Dementia-Friendly Worship

of related interest

Spiritual Care for People Living with Dementia Using Multisensory Interventions
A Practical Guide for Chaplains
Richard Behers
ISBN 978 1 78592 811 6
eISBN 978 1 78450 856 2

A Guide to the Spiritual Dimension of Care for People with Alzheimer's Disease and Related Dementia
More than Body, Brain and Breath
Eileen Shamy
ISBN 978 1 84310 129 1
eISBN 978 1 84642 388 8

Sharing Sensory Stories and Conversations with People with Dementia
A Practical Guide
Joanna Grace
ISBN 978 1 78592 409 5
eISBN 978 1 78450 769 5

Developing a Relational Model of Care for Older People
Creating Environments for Shared Living
James Woodward and Jenny Kartupelis
ISBN 978 1 78592 334 0
eISBN 978 1 78450 655 1

Dementia-Friendly WORSHIP

A Multifaith Handbook for Chaplains, Clergy, and Faith Communities

Edited by
LYNDA EVERMAN and DON WENDORF, Senior Editors

KATHY FOGG BERRY, ROBIN DILL, STEVEN M. GLAZER, RICHARD L. MORGAN, and WILLIAM B. RANDOLPH, Contributing Editors

Foreword by Virginia Biggar

Jessica Kingsley *Publishers*
London and Philadelphia

First published in 2019
by Jessica Kingsley Publishers
73 Collier Street
London N1 9BE, UK
and
400 Market Street, Suite 400
Philadelphia, PA 19106, USA

www.jkp.com

Front cover image source: Michael J. Powell.

Library of Congress Cataloging in Publication Data
A CIP catalog record for this book is available from the Library of Congress

British Library Cataloguing in Publication Data
A CIP catalogue record for this book is available from the British Library

ISBN 978 1 78592 665 5
eISBN 978 1 78592 666 2

Printed and bound by CPI Group (UK) Ltd, Croydon CR0 4YY

SOULS SHINE FORTH: SERVING THE WORSHIP AND SPIRITUAL NEEDS OF PERSONS WITH DEMENTIA

Cover photo by Michael J. Powell, late son of Lynda Everman, taken on a trip with Lynda and Don at Yosemite. People always describe Mike as the most supportive person they'd ever known. His life and this photo mirror the theme of this book: "Souls Shine Forth." When Mike first posted this photo he referenced Shel Silverstein's book *The Giving Tree*, the story of a tree and a little boy who loved each other even into their old age, despite their infirmities and limitations. It ends with the old, weak tree finding it can still give a resting place to the old, tired man to lean on. They were both happy as their souls shone forth in loving care.

In loving memory of our
family members whom we've lost to dementia:

Alvin Joseph Ducote (1913–2001)
Richard A. Everman, Sr. (1940–2012)
Margaret Lyon Morgan (1901–1967)
Ola Gibbs Phillips (1900–1991)
Hazel Oliphant Randolph (1922–2012)
Mary P. Wendorf (1921–2012)
Susan Black Wendorf (1946–2014)
Bill Wunch (1927–2011)
Lois Wunch (1928–2005)

ALL who have been lost to Alzheimer's and related dementias.

These are our loved ones—individuals who have lived good lives and made lasting contributions to their families and communities, individuals who have been taken from us far too soon and too unkindly. We carry your memories with us.

Trish Vradenburg (1946–2017)
Co-Founder, UsAgainstAlzheimer's

Trish's unflinching spirit—her imagination, quick-witted humor, empathy, generosity, and her exceptional tenacity to stop the suffering of others—was captured in her every action and was the hallmark of her relentless advocacy to stop Alzheimer's. We forge ahead in this same spirit.

Contents

WORSHIP SERVICES

Foreword

UsAgainstAlzheimer's is an innovative nonprofit organization committed to stopping this devastating disease by 2020. Powered by our personal experiences and the suffering of millions of families, we press for greater urgency from government, industry, and the scientific community in the quest for an Alzheimer's cure—accomplishing this through effective leadership, collaboration, advocacy, and strategic investments.

We believe that it will take all of "Us" to address this major health challenge. This means cross-sector and community-anchored collaboration around common goals and initiatives. It means being nimble and responsive to partners, communities, policymakers, and the changing healthcare landscape. Collaboration is a core part of the DNA of UsAgainstAlzheimer's and central to our fight for a treatment, prevention and cure.

To achieve this, we work closely with networks of activists and organizations to engage the communities most deeply affected by Alzheimer's through tailored programming and educational outreach efforts. This includes women, African Americans, Latinos, veterans, and people of faith, and we invite all our readers to join us at FaithUnitedAgainstAlzheimers.org.

Faith leaders and communities are on the front lines of the dementia crisis. So often those living with dementia and their families turn first to their faith leaders and communities for solace and support. And many leaders of all faiths are implementing innovative practices and programs to ensure that those affected by Alzheimer's can continue spiritual engagement as valued members of their communities. And as they work to improve quality of life for those living with dementia, faith communities are also leaders in reducing stigma and educating about Alzheimer's, brain health, and clinical trials.

This volume is dedicated in part to UsAgainstAlzheimer's co-founder, Trish Vradenburg, whom we lost in April 2017. In remembering Trish, her brother, Rabbi Michael Lerner, said, "She put her energy into stopping Alzheimer's—a commitment that was actually, I believe, a deeply religious commitment. A commitment to say that when people were saying it's impossible, she would always say, 'No, no, no. It only hasn't happened yet.'"

As Trish wrote, "A cure for Alzheimer's: a fantasy, a wish, an impossible dream—the same words that were said to Galileo, Edison, Curie, Salk, and whoever dreamed up the internet. Yesterday's dream is today's reality."

All of us at UsAgainstAlzheimer's are also indebted to our esteemed contributors representing many faiths and cultural traditions, as well as the critical perspectives of those living with dementia. And I want to express my deep gratitude to our dedicated and passionate team of activist editors who have each cared for loved ones themselves, and who spent countless hours to make their dream of this volume a reality.

Virginia Biggar
Director of Communities
UsAgainstAlzheimer's

Editors' Reflections

This book began as a dream of our friend, Rev. Dr. William Randolph. Will felt inspired to provide resources to chaplains, pastors, and other clergy ministering to persons with dementia on how they could best serve their worship/spiritual needs, given the limitations from their diseases. He wanted this book to honor his late mother, Hazel, who died with Alzheimer's disease. He was only too aware of the lack of available resources, having spent many years working with persons living with dementia as a chaplain himself. The conspiracy to actually produce such a volume was hatched over a five-hour lunch with Will in Nashville in July 2017 at a restaurant not two blocks from where the psychology building used to be during Don's first stint at graduate school at Vanderbilt in 1969. This was also only two blocks from the prayer chapel at Scarrit College where Don and his late wife, Susan, were married in 1972. Forty years later, Don spent years as her caregiver when Susan had vascular dementia and numerous physical impairments from strokes. Don had also overseen the care of his father, Hulen, with mild dementia from Parkinson's disease and his mother, Mary, who died with Alzheimer's disease. So he was excited by Will's ideas and ready to join in the plot.

Lynda, having been the caregiver for her father, Al Ducote, with vascular dementia, and her late husband, Richard Everman, with Alzheimer's, was already a champion advocate for Alzheimer's. She had been a founding member of ActivistsAgainstAlzheimer's, ClergyAgainstAlzheimer's, and WomenAgainstAlzheimer's. Moreover, on behalf of ClergyAgainstAlzheimer's, she had already co-edited *Seasons of Caring: Meditations for Alzheimer's and Dementia Caregivers* (Potts *et al.* 2014). In fact, it was Don's contribution to that book, "Painted Bits of Bark and Stone and Tin" (a tribute to Susan), from his book to help caregivers with their emotional struggles (*Caregiver Carols: A Musical,*

Emotional Memoir (Wendorf 2014)), that had brought Don and Lynda together in the first place. That collaboration resulted in our marriage, and California girl Lynda moved to Don's home in Birmingham. Together, Don and Lynda had also helped edit several books by Rev. Dr. Richard Morgan. So, having only done a modest amount of book editing ourselves and with neither of us being clergy or having the slightest notion of how to actually do this ministering, we felt totally capable of taking on this project! We eagerly joined the conspiracy. Mostly we had our *feelings* to go on: deep empathy for the people experiencing these dreadful diseases and intense concern for their care partners who give their lives to providing the most loving care possible. We had both been ministered to in incredibly loving ways by clergy and faith communities during our caregiving and this was a chance to "pay it forward."

So, we bravely began to assemble our team of editorial experts to help us formulate the content, find contributors, and polish submissions into the book you now are reading. Rev. Dr. Will Randolph, who at that point was still with Discipleship Ministries, a division of the United Methodist Church, is an expert on aging and spirituality and passionate about serving the spiritual needs of Baby Boomers and older adults. Eventually, Will left this job and returned to his earlier career as a chaplain in senior living centers, moving back to Pennsylvania to work at Longwood Presbyterian Senior Care in Verona. Will had been introduced to us by his mentor, also our dear friend and a co-editor of *Seasons of Caring: Meditations for Alzheimer's and Dementia Caregivers*, Rev. Dr. Richard Morgan. Richard was quick to be drafted from his home at Redstone Highlands Senior Living Community near Pittsburgh, Pennsylvania, where he was living in a continuing care facility with his wife Alice Ann. Richard is the author of some 20-plus books on spirituality and aging, and a "retired" pastor who, at age 88, was still functioning as a volunteer chaplain, leading dementia support groups. Now at 89, he continues to inspire us with his blog, "Notes Near Ninety," that he shares with family and friends.

Richard and Will brought Robin Dill onto the editorial team. Both of Robin's parents, Bill and Lois Wunch, had dementia and she had been a contributor to *Seasons*; but, she was mostly recruited for her years of experience directing an incredibly compassionate respite care program. Robin wrote about it in her book *Walking with Grace Revised: Tools for Implementing and Launching a Congregational Respite Program* (2016), a tremendous resource for congregations wanting to begin their own respite programs. She has helped start a number of respite programs in the Southeastern U.S. Also enlisted for her excellent book and training program in ministering to persons with dementia was Rev. Kathy Fogg Berry. Kathy is a chaplain for memory care at Westminster Canterbury Richmond (VA). Her practical, but exquisitely loving, book and DVD *When Words Fail: Practical Ministry to People with Dementia and Their Caregivers* (2018) are what we recommend for those just starting to serve the needs of dementia patients.

Lynda originally met editor Rabbi Steven Glazer through Ian Kremer of the LEAD (Leaders Engaged on Alzheimer's Disease) Coalition who recommended him as another founder when she was organizing ClergyAgainstAlzheimer's. He later worked with her in editing *Seasons*. He is a giant in interfaith understanding and advocacy as well as with Alzheimer's, although he has not been a care partner with someone with dementia. However, he took care of his late wife, Andrea, who had serious medical problems and he is a most devoted and empathetic champion for Alzheimer's efforts and other caregivers. He was actually a rabbi in Birmingham while Don was also living there and working as a psychologist. But, as is the case with another of her co-editors and a contributor to this book, Dr. Danny Potts of Tuscaloosa (who knew Don's employer and sang in choral groups with him), Don had to marry Lynda to get to know both Steve and Danny. Don was a mentor for a family therapist whose friend was a close friend of Danny and that's how Don was encouraged to send Lynda his piece for *Seasons*. Our complex connections are amazingly "coincidental" and ultimately meaningful. It's a funny world, but one of the best things about writing this book has been all the connections we've learned we have or have now formed with some of the most caring, creative and generous people out there, all of whom share a profound compassion for persons afflicted by dementias and their loved ones. Is there some other plot "out there" to make us all friends and collaborators?

Although not as heavily involved in content editing, the final member of our team is Ginny Biggar, who is our rock, not to mention the staff rock as UsAgainstAlzheimer's Director of Communities. Ginny provides all the administrative support and reality checks anyone could ask for. Moreover, she is always patient and open-minded when we propose some other wild scheme for the book or our Dementia-Friendly Faith Initiative or plot some new promotion for Lynda's other big passion: the Alzheimer's Semipostal Stamp that raises research funds for the National Institutes of Health. Ginny's faith in us is reassuring and very supportive.

Once into this scheme, our plot thickened considerably and the book has evolved beyond our initial vision and expectations. It begins with a faith-infused section on what dementia involves, how this affects spiritual and worship needs and capacities, and what clergy can do about it. Leading this is dear friend and deep man of faith, Dr. Danny Potts, a Tuscaloosa neurologist. He and his family have helped care for nine family members with dementia, including his father, Lester, who found out at Caring Days Adult Day Care Center that he had a gift for painting despite his Alzheimer's, a gift that transformed his life and his ability to relate once more to his family. Lynda and Don participate each semester in Danny's Bringing Art to Life program there, with Don performing music and Lynda giving her personalized quilts to participants. Danny is an accomplished vocalist, poet, and photographer, and his article seems like the only medical treatise we've ever read that was written in theological poetry.

> A crucial theme here, echoed throughout the book, is that in spite of the cognitive and other limitations imposed by dementias, the essence of the person, their core, their *soul*, is still there, very much alive, and able to be ministered to and meaningfully connected with, given the right training, expectations, openness, and resources. That's what we want this book to address, and an outstanding group of contributors have shared their expertise and caring to make this happen.

Following this introductory section is Don's favorite section: articles written by people who have diagnoses of dementia. We are honored to give these courageous people a voice here. They relate their experiences, how their dementia affects them and their needs and their abilities to participate in worship, and how they would like clergy to understand, relate to, and serve them. One of these, Rev. Cynthia Huling Hummel, is still working part-time as a pastor. Another, Greg O'Brien, has had a distinguished national career as a journalist and author. Imagine how intimidating it has been to presume to offer editorial assistance to Greg. Fortunately, he is a most accepting, kind man, with a fabulous sense of humor. Oh, to be able to write like he has…and *still does*! These "voices of dementia" authors have repeatedly brought home to us one of the most important themes that have emerged in this book:

> It is so easy to focus on what people with dementia can no longer do; it is of utmost importance, not to mention inspirational, transformative, and redemptive, to observe what they *still can do*. And *are doing!!!!!*

The heart, and soul, of the book is the middle section, in which people of very different backgrounds and expertise and faith traditions share their vast store of experience and knowledge with us. They get right down to the essentials of how best to relate to people with dementia and their worship/spiritual needs, whether that be on a one-to-one pastoral visit or in a small group in a memory care unit, or within an entire congregational worship setting. Despite all their differences, we were repeatedly struck by the similarities in the wisdom these people shared. It was important to us that the book be interfaith, like the world we live in and the population clergy serve. We are honored to present Christian, Jewish, Muslim, Sikh Dharma, Buddhist, and Native American perspectives.

> Among the many themes emerging in this middle section were how vital it is to use expressive arts, especially music, in worship and how one can and must enter the world of the person with dementia to share spiritual connection and worship experiences.

The last main section has several articles in which authors explore some of the ways clergy can expand their congregational response to persons living with dementia and their family members. This might include respite care, assistance to caregivers, expressive arts programs, advocacy, a more easily navigated physical space, compiling resources, support groups, legal advice, exercise activities, or meals: things that keep them meaningfully involved as part of their faith community. This is the section on becoming "dementia-friendly" faith communities: how to do it and why it is so important. And not only "dementia-friendly" but "dementia *active*." Perhaps the most significant theme that emerged here was one that touched us so deeply: *not only can we discover ways to truly provide ministry for persons with dementia, we can minister with them, as spiritual partners in connecting with each other, our faith communities and God.* Not just "*for*" but "*with.*" We can find ways these souls can still contribute to and be a part of a worship community and, in the process, *they can provide us with spiritual connection, enrichment, nourishment, and growth.* Our central theme has been *"souls shine forth."*

Lynda Everman and Don Wendorf
Senior Editors

References

Dill, R. (2016) *Walking with Grace Revised: Tools for Implementing and Launching a Congregational Respite Program*. iUniverse.

Fogg Berry, K. (2018) *When Words Fail: Practical Ministry to People with Dementia and Their Caregivers*. Grand Rapids, MI: Kregel Publications.

Potts, D.C., Everman, L., Glazer, S.M., Morgan, R.L., and Wallack, M. (eds) (2014) *Seasons of Caring: Meditations for Alzheimer's and Dementia Caregivers*. CreateSpace Independent Publishing Platform.

Wendorf, D. (2014) *Caregiver Carols: A Musical, Emotional Memoir*. CreateSpace Independent Publishing Platform.

INTRODUCTION TO DEMENTIA-FRIENDLY WORSHIP

Introduction: Souls Shine Forth

Serving the Worship/Spiritual Needs of Persons with Dementia

Daniel C. Potts, MD, FAAN (Presbyterian Church, USA)

How could this be? He hadn't spoken in weeks. His face, expressionless, except for the tears that seemed to upwell at deep moments of connection or beauty, saying more than words could ever express.

> Then I shall bow, in humble adoration, and there proclaim, "My God, how great Thou art!"

Yet, as we gathered there at hospice, those who loved him—both blood kin and others drawn together in spirit through the kinship of faith—he still was able to sing the words which had become life itself for him through the years. When the mind has lost its capacity to formulate and express thoughts...

> Then sings my soul...

> The Spirit helps us in our weakness; for we do not know how to pray as we ought, but that very Spirit intercedes with sighs too deep for words. (Romans 8.26, *New Revised Standard Version*)

My father, Lester E. Potts, Jr., a man of deep faith and integrity, passed away from complications related to Alzheimer's disease in 2007. A neurologist and his only child, I coped poorly with both the reality of the disease, and the finality of its effects. Reaching the end of my own inner resources a few years after his death, I must have resembled someone at late-stage, though my disease was characterized by the blank stare of self-sufficiency and the rising fever of resentment.

Yet there was the searching, the surrender, the wordless prayer...

> Prayer begins at the edge of emptiness. (Heschel 2005)

Like others living with dementia of any kind, my father experienced not only the loss of memory, but also the loss of the ability to express himself through spoken language, a condition termed *aphasia*. This inability to communicate verbally contributes to the isolation often experienced both by the ones living with dementia and their care partners.

Persons living with dementia, especially early on, may be cognizant of some of the changes that are occurring, and may avoid contact with others. Care partners may draw back from social settings because of the commitment of time and responsibility inherent in their new role, concern about what others might think, or a desire to shield their loved one from the embarrassment or shame they fear might arise in awkward encounters.

Likewise, well-meaning friends and loved ones stay away, not knowing what to say or how to interact. Many, unconsciously influenced by the stigma society has against those with cognitive impairment, may question the benefits of visiting someone who has forgotten them or, they assume, may forget any uplifts that were experienced during the time of the visit. Science has shown, however, that both positive and negative emotional effects may persist for persons living with dementia for hours after the encounters have ended, even if there is no memory of the visits themselves.

The burgeoning field of interpersonal neurobiology explores the neuroscience of relationships and attachment and how they affect the brain's plasticity, or ability to change throughout life. For instance, it has now been shown that being in an enriching environment of supportive relationships, where creativity, mental and physical exercise, and novel experiences are fostered, the brains of even the elderly show beneficial changes that promote resiliency and well-being. By the same token, being deprived of such stimulation is detrimental to the structure and function of the brain.

Of all the losses associated with dementia, I believe *the greatest loss is that of relationship*. Yet a sense of relationship is vital to the integrity of the self.

> We are here to awaken from our illusion of separateness. (Thich Nhat Hanh, Buddhist monk and teacher, from Stanley, Loy, and Dorje 2009)

What fuels the toxicity of this stigma, of this pulling away? I believe it is our failure to recognize and honor the inherent personhood of every human being, regardless of conditions or circumstances. The loss of personhood does not follow from the loss of cognitive abilities. I strongly understand personhood as being imparted, and therefore inviolate, unfading, even unending. And certainly not lessened by any disease.

If I do not hold such a view of personhood, then I am apt to regard those who experience cognitive loss as "less than," negatively biasing my treatment of them, and my expectations of being able to form or maintain relationships with them. This amounts to a judgment…a judgment in favor of dementia, and against the human spirit.

Yet we do not exist within a vacuum. Ancient wisdom and spiritual traditions teach that we exist in and through relationship, ever seeking such unity. So, as in a mirror, we see that our own bias and judgment reflect upon ourselves. Are we to let our notions about dementia, or any condition that might be labeled a "disability," quench the inner flame that burns more brightly in the oxygen-rich presence of others?

> The sacred flame of your inner shrine is constantly bright. The experience of unity is the fulfillment of human endeavors. (*The Rig Veda*, trans. Doniger 2005)

My father found this soul fire through the expressive arts, and by being together with others in the act of creating. Watercolors, coupled with music, movement, literature, drama, reminiscence—and the supportive milieu of those who believed in him and met him in his world—enabled Dad to share the story of Lester—who he was, still, despite the disease—and brought us back into a meaningful relationship with him. The resulting re-union bound together the edges of cuts laid deep by the hands of Alzheimer's. The Latin, "religio," root word of religion, means "to bind." Dad's new religion was artistic expression, though in truth it was the same "old time religion" that had been such an essential part of his life, morphed into a different kind of worship experience—one that enabled him to be himself.

Faith and worship had always taken its place in the center of my father's life and that of his family. Life-long Methodists, my parents were introduced by a Methodist minister at a revival. When later asked by my mother what would have happened to their relationship had she not been Methodist, Dad quipped, "We wouldn't have had one." And yet, his son fell for a Presbyterian! I think old Papa has forgiven me. He did love my dear Ellen.

To the observer, it appears even one's expression and practice of faith is not spared from the ravages of dementia. We already have mentioned the isolating effects of the loss of communication associated with aphasia, one of the cardinal features of Alzheimer's disease, and common with other dementias such as vascular, frontotemporal, and Lewy Body. One could see how short-term memory loss, or *amnesia,* could negatively impact the ability to worship in a traditional sense, as well. The hippocampus, the primary brain region in which the processing and filing of new information associated with making memories takes place, also is involved in interpreting spatial relationships. This region of the brain is affected early and severely in Alzheimer's disease, and contributes a great deal to the associated disability. Commonly visited spaces begin to look different, often leading to agitation and an urge to physically move to a place of familiarity, which can be disruptive in a worship service.

Disinhibition often develops in persons living with dementia, and can lead to inappropriate behaviors such as vocalization, wandering, or unwanted touching in worship services and other social settings. In my father's case, as the ministers recessed down the aisle after the benediction, Dad would often stand up and block their exit for a firm handshake or his characteristic pronouncement: "I'm proud of you." Thankfully, his ministers knew this to be an expression of the warmth and richness of his character, rather than something threatening. Nevertheless, it was disruptive.

People living with dementia may be unable to control their emotions at certain times, tending to mirror the emotional tone sensed in their environment. This is the reason care partners are taught to guard against any expression of agitation, irritability, or anger in themselves, as these will likely be mirrored in persons living with dementia. It is possible that the tone of certain worship environments, especially if unfamiliar, might be emotionally misinterpreted, leading to agitation or other behaviors in persons living with dementia.

Care partners and worship leaders should learn to identify non-verbal expressions of anxiety or agitation, and try to redirect through music, prayer, gentle touch if welcomed, pleasant facial expressions, etc. Interpersonal interactions always should occur face to face at eye level, clearly, slowly, and with good volume and enunciation, asking open-ended questions, and allowing individuals time to express themselves uncorrected or without having words chosen for them unless they have requested help. All care partner behavior should strive to be upbuilding and characterized by compassion, gentleness, and validation, with redirection if needed.

Returning to the field of interpersonal neurobiology, certain behaviors that may be elements of faith-based practice, such as meditation and mindfulness, promote beneficial changes in brain structure and function which have been associated with a sense of well-being and calm. For instance, activity in the amygdala, the part of the brain's limbic system associated with certain emotions related to survival, particularly fear, is modulated in a top-down fashion primarily by structures located in the frontal cortex. Meditation and mindfulness activities enhance the function and bolster the structure of the pathways modulating function in the amygdala and other parts of the limbic system, thereby enabling greater control over emotions, lowering the likelihood of unchecked fear or anxiety reactions.

In addition to the cognitive effects of dementia, there are physical manifestations that may get overlooked. Balance and gait usually are affected progressively, so that persons with dementia are apt to fall, posing a safety risk to themselves or others. Loss of urinary bladder or bowel control creates difficulties, both with incontinence, and with problems interpreting the urge to use the facilities. Furthermore, persons with dementia may forget they have used the bathroom and attempt to go one or more times during a worship service.

Communion, a sacrament in the Christian tradition and of vital importance in the life of faith, may become difficult to negotiate for persons living with dementia. *Apraxia*, or the inability to execute a voluntary motor movement despite having the strength to do so, may render someone unable to take the bread, to hold the cup, to kneel, etc. Activities thus may need to be broken down into their root elements, with visual and tactile cues and reinforcement given to accomplish more complex tasks. Because coordination and control of the swallowing muscles often is progressively lost (or lost suddenly as the result of a stroke or cerebral hemorrhage), one may not be able to take the communion elements without coughing or overtly choking, or without being coached through the swallowing process by someone who is knowledgeable in such matters.

Agnosia, or the inability to cortically process sensory information leading to a lack of recognition of objects, persons, sounds, shapes, or smells, is also a cardinal feature of Alzheimer's, and is present in other dementias, as well. While perhaps not appearing to have as much of a negative effect as some of the other manifestations of dementia, when considered from the position of a person living with the disease, this may have a profound impact. The sensory environment in many worship spaces contributes strongly to the experience, whether through the smell of incense, recited liturgies, prayers, or mantras, sacred dances or postures, the presence of nature, the power of icons, windows, or other religious symbols, or the singing of chants or hymns. Some feel they are ushered into the realm of the sacred through experiential accompaniments to worship such as these, yet inability to process them might lessen what is felt inwardly.

> To encounter the sacred is to be alive at the deepest center of human existence. (Momaday, N. Scott n.d.)

These limitations considered, still, those of us who have been care partners, or who have interacted for any length of time with persons living with dementia, know that there remains a presence, deportment, vitality, and integrity of personhood that may be perceived if we are willing to surrender to the phenomenon of being fully alive and undefended in the mutuality of the present moment. That is, if we are brave enough to enter the deep and silent spaces, both luminous and dark, where true relationship occurs.

> Let us pause in silence, amid clamor and confusion, hurries and worries, fear and frustration. (from a speech by Rev. William Sinkford, President, Unitarian Universalist Association)

Toward the end of my father's life, after he had transitioned to an inpatient hospice facility, ministers and staff from both my parents' and my family's churches asked if they could come and offer communion. When Mother told me about this, we both shared a moment of profound gratitude at such a gift. To me, there could be no greater representation of meeting him in his current reality, of honoring his faith that had held through the storms of Alzheimer's. And to my surprise, he was able to participate despite the apraxia, aphasia, agnosia, and amnesia that characterized his condition, taking the bread and grape juice from the polished cup and tray.

> There is a polish for everything that takes away rust and the polish for the heart is the remembrance of God. (Muhammed, quoted in Brown 2009)

How, then, do we provide opportunities through which persons living with dementia may have meaningful experiences of worship? We must create safe and supportive environments for the expression of personhood through enabling creativity, engaging imagination and the senses, and sharing of stories in community, whether in a gathering of two or 200 (though in the context of dementia, intimate settings may be preferable).

All of us have life stories to share. Dementia, through its effects on verbal expression, can adversely impact the ability to share stories. Nevertheless, faith, or the search for it, weaves its way through our narrative. We must let ourselves be led into worship by persons living with dementia, trusting them to guide us through the sacred stories to those shared spaces of familiarity, community, love, expression, and relationship. Once we see the candles of that inner sanctuary, we must be willing to go there, with all our accompaniments, and worship with them in a language all of us can speak—the language of authenticity, vulnerability, presence, wonder, gratitude, compassion, and love.

> I will praise the Lord as long as I live. I will sing praises to my God with my dying breath. (Psalm 146.2; *New Living Translation* (*NLT*))

The gathering itself, whether by one or many, is a communal prayer, a calling to a higher plane. On my father's final day on earth, as the last friends and family began to leave for the evening, Dad moved his unfocused stare to a spot near the corner of the ceiling, there maintaining his gaze with intense clarity for over an hour. Expecting no response, I asked him what he was looking at. He turned directly toward me with the most piercing expressivity I had seen on his face in years, and calmly said, "My Mama."

Perhaps we can join in this "communion of saints" through our nearness, our silence, our presence in experiences of shared worship.

At my father's memorial service, our family's minister, Dr. Charles Durham, shared these words:

> Faith is deeply implanted, deeply rooted, and nothing can ever separate us from the love of God. Even in his most difficult times, Lester Potts could still pray the Lord's Prayer, and mouth the prayers of the blessing. As this family gathered round and sang the Lord's praises and hymns, that man of faith would mouth them right along with them. And so, we know, beyond any shadow of a doubt, that [God's] righteousness goes to His children's children.

As I was reminded by theologian and dementia care partner, Dr. James Houston, who was discussing his role as memory-bearer for his wife, Rita:

> We are eternally remembered. This, then, is projected back into our current situation. Rita, my dear, let me be memory to you.

In worship experiences with persons who are living with dementia, we, too, can be memory-bearers, reminding them that God's righteousness extends even unto them.

The following pages contain a double portion of wisdom, heart, experience, and scholarship regarding the creation of meaningful worship opportunities for persons living with dementia, opportunities which honor personhood, story, imagination, relationships, and God, as God may be understood. The authors fully acknowledge the effects of dementia upon individuals, families, and care partners. Yet they do not give dementia the final word. Instead, focusing on remaining strengths, with deference to persons living with dementia themselves as ushers into that sacred gathering place, they follow with their prayers, voices, instruments, elements, and, most of all, their stories and their hearts.

The relationships themselves, with self, others, God, and all that exists in the sacrament of the present moment, fully lived and fully shared, have the power to transform and to heal.

Thus quickened, we may be able to create a culture of compassion for persons living with dementia, along with their care partners and loved ones. Perhaps, by helping them connect to themselves, the people around them, their faith, and their sense of the Divine presence through worship experiences, we may empower their souls to shine forth in beauty and clarity through the dark clouds of dementia.

In so doing, may our own souls shine forth with theirs, aflame with the eternal light of Love shared in unity of the spirit, for the good of us all.

References

Brown, J.A.C. (2009) *Hadith: Muhammad's Legacy in the Medieval and Modern World (Foundations of Islam).* London: Oneworld Publications.

Doniger, W. (trans.) (2005) *The Rig Veda.* New York: Penguin Classics.

Heschel, A.J. (2005) *The Sabbath.* New York: Farrar, Straus and Giroux.

Momaday, N. Scott (n.d.) 'Address to the United Nations at the "Cry of the Earth" Gathering in November 1993, the Gathering of Indigenous Peoples of the Americas at the United Nations.' Retrieved from www.wisdomoftheelders.org/un-address-n-scott-momaday on November 02, 2018.

Stanley, J., Loy, D.R., and Dorje, G. (eds) (2009) *A Buddhist Response to the Climate Emergency.* Somerville, MA: Wisdom Publications.

Worshi Adaptations

Rev. Linn Possell (United Church of Christ)

As clergy we know that the spirit transcends all things and that people living with dementia can have a beautiful quality of life when we believe in that possibility and allow them the grace and freedom to be. While dementia presents challenges, the spirit remains whole and beautiful, just as God has created it.

When thinking about preparing a worship experience for someone living with brain change, there are a few things to consider. Regardless of what spiritual path someone travels, these considerations remain the same because they have to do with the changes that are happening in the brain and how people take in information. In this section I will focus on four things to consider: pace, vision, language, and sensory motor abilities. We all know that people living with dementia can experience the divine in many ways, and one is through worship; there are some very important adjustments that we can make that will enable someone to experience worship through end of life with dementia.

I invite you to think about a portion of worship as I review specific changes in the brain and offer adaptations as you consider what you might do to help those to whom you minister.

Pace

People living with dementia need a longer time to take in information, try to make sense of that information, and then respond. When I was learning counseling, I was told that it takes about 21 seconds for someone to process and respond to a question in counseling. As we practiced our counseling, we were taught to count to 21, and then if the person did not respond we could ask another question. This was all to get us comfortable with the silence that can happen while a person thinks about a response. If you take the time to count out 21 seconds, you will see that it seems like a long time. People living with dementia need more time to process information. A good way to be sure you are allowing time for them to process information is to wait seven to 12 seconds before you offer another prompt. This is because while the gray matter in the brain that holds information is shrinking and dying, the white matter that is the wiring or connections to the places that hold information is also affected. Pace is important: when reading a text or offering communion, give the person living with dementia *time* to take in, process, and respond.

Vision

People living with dementia experience significant vision changes. In the earliest stage of dementia, usually before diagnosis, people have limited peripheral vision as if they are seeing through a scuba mask. If you put your hands up to block out your peripheral vision and touch your little fingers and thumbs together, this is the vision someone in the early stage of dementia has. In middle stages, the vision is like looking through binoculars, and by the late stage, vision is monocular. Therefore you will need to make sure that you and what you are using for worship is provided in their visual field. They may not see the entire worship space, altar, or even hymnal. The other vision change that happens is that people can lose the ability to know what an object does or is used for and therefore may need assistance and guidance when given items during worship. If someone seems to be confused as to how to use an item or participate in some way, make sure that you are in their visual field and give them visual cues such as demonstrating how to use an item. This will allow the person dignity as well as helping them be successful in their participation.

Language

We have language in both temporal lobes of our brain. In the left temporal, we have word finding, comprehension, and vocabulary. This is the lobe that is affected by dementia. The right temporal lobe, however, is not affected by dementia. In this lobe we retain social chit chat: "Hi, how are you? I'm fine, and you? How's it going? Not bad," and so on. This social chit chat can cause us to think that someone understands more than they do. We can get surprised by someone who can use social chit chat but then has trouble with the content of speech. However, social chit chat provides a way for us to stay connected and engaged during the disease. Another form of speech that is retained is profanity, racial slurs, and sex words, especially if someone did not use them on a regular basis. This can cause some anxiety and misunderstanding from family members and congregations and requires some education that this is not coming from the person but from the disease and that people living with dementia are always doing the best they can. Knowing this bit of information about the right temporal lobe helps those of us around people living with dementia to grant them some grace. The blessing of the right temporal lobe is that rhythm, music, poetry, and prayer are located here as well. Someone living with dementia will be able to sing old familiar songs and say old familiar prayers long into the disease. Therefore, use old songs, prayers, and rituals that have been memorized to help people living with dementia stay engaged.

Sensory motor

People living with dementia usually will lose the ability to manipulate objects at some point, and when this occurs you will want to remember that while they can no longer use their hands for tasks, they still will respond to gentle soothing touch. Holding someone's hand can be an experience of the divine; it is comforting and soothing and can let someone feel God's presence.

Taking all of these brain changes into mind, when using an old familiar song for the worship experience, for example, consider these things:

- accentuate the rhythm of the song; have enough of an intro that the person can recognize it; and make sure that the pace is not too fast
- use an old song that is short and repetitive, or use only the most familiar verses
- use a single song sheet with large words or a picture that has a familiar symbol that corresponds to the song and present the sheet in the person's field of vision in such a way that it does not startle them
- clap, sway, or use body movement so the person feels the rhythm of the song.

Continuing to Hear the Voice

A Reflection

Rabbi Cary D. Kozberg, MAHL, DD (Jewish)

> The voice of the Lord is in power… (Psalm 29.4; *JPS Hebrew-English TANAKH*)

Expounding on this verse, the ancient rabbinic Sages taught that it refers to the experience of the Israelites at Mount Sinai when God gave them the Ten Commandments. They point out that the specific phrase "in power" refers to God's unique power to communicate to each and every person who was present at that singular event, *each according to his/her own individual abilities*:

- the men heard it according to their abilities, and the women heard it according to their abilities
- the wise heard it according to their abilities, and the simple heard it according to their abilities
- likewise, the young heard it according to their abilities, and the elderly heard it according to their abilities.

(Midrash Song of Songs, Rabbah 5.16 and Midrash Exodus Rabbah 5.9 and 29.4)

What is their point? Why emphasize that every person at Sinai heard God's Voice, each in his/her own unique way and regardless of gender, intellectual capacity, or age? Is it not a given that God can do whatever God desires? Perhaps they wanted to remind us that *when God addresses us, we hear the Voice not just with our minds, but more importantly with our souls.*

Certainly, anyone who has spent a significant amount of time with individuals who have dementia comes to learn this truth. Anyone who has spent a significant amount of time *relating* to such individuals will affirm that dementia may indeed "steal the mind," but it does not steal the heart, or the soul, or the spirit. Contrary to conventional wisdom, dementia may take away a person's cognition and memory, but it most certainly does *not* take away their humanity.

One person who comes to mind whenever I rehearse this truth is a man I will call Joe. A life-long observant Jew, Joe was a resident in the long-term care facility where I was a chaplain for over 25 years. As his dementia worsened, he lost most of his short-term memory, was often incontinent, and needed regular assistance with everyday activities. Still, despite his cognitive deficits, Joe retained remarkable social skills, greeting me every Friday afternoon (as we prepared for the Sabbath) with a warm handshake, a friendly smile, and the same enthusiastic greeting, "*Rabbi, it's time to talk to the Boss!*"

To be sure, he often forgot the words to blessings he had recited thousands of times, and offered answers that often didn't fit the questions he was asked. Nevertheless, despite the cognitive loss he had sustained, Joe was one of the most *spiritually alive* people I have ever known.

Individuals like Joe highlight what our Judeo-Christian tradition teaches about reverence for God and how His love for us echoes in how we treat people like Joe. Scripture commands us to "Stand up in the presence of the aged, show respect for the elderly and revere your God. I am the LORD" (Leviticus 19.32). Significantly, this verse does not mention ensuring that our elders are fed or clothed well, or are housed in "state of the art" residential venues. Rather, it focuses on our "showing respect"—paying attention to, and not ignoring, them. Indeed, because it is so easy to ignore them and not notice them—because they are so often "invisible" to the rest of society. Scripture reminds us that there is always *Someone* noticing. Hence, the connection of this commandment to reverence for God.

Significantly, the above-quoted verse is followed by: "If a stranger sojourns in your land, you shall do him no wrong...you shall love him as yourself, for you were strangers in the land of Egypt" (Leviticus 19.33). The juxtaposition of these two verses is, I believe, significant: Scripture seems to be emphasizing that we must guard against treating our older adults as if they were strangers—and especially those whose cognitive decline make them speak and act in ways that are most "strange" and incomprehensible to us.

Moreover, connecting the commandment about "showing respect to the elderly" with that of "loving the stranger" teaches us about loving those with cognitive decline. Love of the stranger is an *unconditional* love: it means loving a person that you don't know, someone with whom you have no history, and therefore someone you don't necessarily trust.

Therefore, it is a love that is risky, because one doesn't know if the recipient is "worthy."

And yet, loving the stranger reflects the kind of unconditional, unearned love shown by God Himself to us, without regard to our "worthiness":

> It is not because you are the most numerous of peoples that the Lord set His heart on you and chose you...but it was because the Lord loved you... (Deuteronomy 7.7)

> For God so loved the world that He gave His only begotten son... (John 3.16)

Thus, it may be that our loving those with cognitive impairment, the "strangers in our midst," is not so much about their worthiness as receivers of that love, but more about increasing our worthiness as *givers* of that love. Folks with dementia automatically are worthy of God's love, but that love is made manifest only when we choose to unconditionally impart it.

And if those with dementia do indeed continue to hear the Voice not so much with their minds but with their souls, that love is made manifest when we create and sustain their spiritual connections, including making worship experiences more accessible to them. Indeed, for those who have participated in religious worship for most of their lives, listening to familiar prayers and Scripture passages, hearing hymns long embedded in their long-term memories (and spontaneously perking up to sing them, even when they no longer express themselves in other ways!) usually proves to be a much-needed boon to their spiritual, and overall, well-being. Whether a person says the blessing over the Sabbath candles, accepts the communion cup, holds the rosary and automatically recites the "Hail Mary," or merely taps a foot even while being "out of it" in a wheelchair, the souls of such individuals remain "response-*able*," despite their cognitive losses; they still hear the Voice and respond according to their own unique abilities.

Moreover, their hearing the Voice not only affirms their own personal relationship with God, but also affirms their life-long relationship with their respective faith communities, even when members of those communities may have forgotten them. This is a crucial point for those of us who care about their overall well-being. We who still affirm people with dementia to still be *people*, created in the Divine image, must also affirm those relationships, even when they no longer can. It is *we* who must remember they remain members of our faith communities, and are by no means strangers to be ignored and disenfranchised. When we help them sustain their spiritual connections, when we help make worship more accessible to them, we affirm that even when they have forgotten, even when others have forgotten them—God never will forget hem.

> Be careful with an old person who has lost his memory because of his troubles, since it is said that both the second set of tablets (of the Ten Commandments) and the broken tablets that Moses shattered were housed together in the Holy Ark. (Talmud Tractate Brakhot, 8b)

As we strive to help them continue to hear and respond to the Voice that still calls to them, may this teaching, also from the ancient rabbinic Sages, remind us of the sanctity of our efforts, as well as the abiding sanctity of those who benefit from them.

VOICES OF PERSONS LIVING WITH DEMENTIA

Editors' Note

This section is very meaningful and special to us as the articles are written by persons who are actually living with dementia themselves. We are presenting their works as close to how they were written as possible, including some rather idiosyncratic spellings, phrasings, word usages, and sentence structures. It is so easy to see what people have lost because of their dementia; it is of utmost importance to us to focus on what they still can do and are doing. These articles are their voices, and we want them to really be *in their voices*. It is how we honor, support, respect, and admire our brothers and sisters struggling to live as full lives as possible. It also gives them the opportunity to use their own experiences to minister to you and the lives you touch. This is in the spirit of addressing their spiritual/worship needs *with* them, not just *for* them.

From Death to Life

My Alzheimer's Journey

Rev. Dr. Cynthia Huling Hummel (Presbyterian Church, USA)

The Cemetery

I was trying not to hyperventilate, but I was on the verge of a total meltdown. I glanced down at the clock. There was no way I was going to arrive on time for the gravesite service. The clock was tick-tick-ticking away and I could picture the family members dressed in black and waiting anxiously. I was so distraught, I couldn't even remember the name of the family and even worse—the name of the deceased. I knew that it was three letters. Was it Bob? Sam? Ben? (Why couldn't I remember it?) I pulled over and called the church, hoping that my secretary, Margo, would pick up the phone and rescue me. Three rings. Four rings. Five rings...then voice mail. The tears were streaming down my face. Why couldn't I find the cemetery?

One of the symptoms of Alzheimer's disease is confusion about time and place.

The Florist

I decided to call a local florist for directions. "Marvin, it's Pastor Cynthia. Can you tell me how to get to the Waverly Cemetery?" He started to laugh. "This is a joke, right? No, I can tell you're DEAD serious. Haha." Trust me—I was not in the mood for Marvin's burial humor. I just wanted to get to the cemetery. Marvin stayed on the phone with me—served as my "gps" and got me to the cemetery—he even mentioned that he had delivered flowers earlier for the family of JIM Smith (Thank you, JESUS, Mary & Marv!!) I was going to be late but, at least, I had the name of the deceased. I was shaken to my core by the ordeal, but I somehow pulled myself together, grabbed my funeral book, got out of my car and walked over to the family. The funeral director introduced me and whispered to me later—"I thought for sure you were a no-show. Why were you so late? I was about ready to plant Jim myself." I apologized and made up some reason why I was late—but I didn't tell him the truth—that I was lost and couldn't find the cemetery and that by the way—my brain was dying too.

Sometimes a person with Alzheimer's disease may forget where she is or how she got there. She may have trouble navigating and may get lost.

Where Did My Memories Go?

Fred stopped by my office on a Wednesday morning. He dropped off some canned goods for the food pantry and told me how much he liked my sermon on Sunday. Instead of being pleased, I started to panic. What had I preached on? I had no idea! Nada—but guessed it had something to do with Jesus and so I asked him what part of the message had resonated with him. He told me that he really liked hearing the story about the family. My mind was racing. What family? What happened to them? As soon as Fred left, I turned on my computer and searched for the sermon. Honestly—it was scary—because it was like reading it for the first time. Why couldn't I remember writing it? Preaching it? I opened a text book to check a reference. There were notes in the margin. I had obviously read the book—but could not remember anything about it. Moreover, I could read the words on the page—but I didn't know what they meant. What was wrong with my brain? I was scared!

One of the most common signs of Alzheimer's is memory loss, especially forgetting recently learned information. Others include: forgetting important dates or events; asking for the same information over and over; increasingly needing to rely on memory aids (e.g. reminder notes or electronic devices) or family members for things they used to handle on their own.

Times of Testing

I sat nervously in the neuropsychologist's office sipping hot coffee and trying to calm my nerves. I hated the 4 hour long neuro-psych tests (and this was my third round in three years). The tester smiled and tried to put me at ease: "I'm going to read you a list of words and I want you to remember them." My mind went blank as I tried to recall the words. I felt so pathetic. She continued in her way too perky voice: "Now I'm going to tell you a story and have you repeat it back to me with as many details as possible." I tried to reconstruct the story: Mrs. Smith of 123 Main Street (or was it Mrs. Main, on Smith Street? I couldn't be sure) had three children—or was it three cats? I couldn't remember...and on and on the torture went. The doctor came in and sat down to observe the testing. The last thing I wanted or needed was a witness to my stupidity. I was mortified. She said, "You're a pastor—with a doctorate in ministry. Can you name the books of the Old Testament?" My heart was racing and I echoed her question: "The books of the Old Testament? Uhhh. Okay." I started slowly: "Genesis, Exodus, Leviticus..." and my mind totally blanked. The books had evaporated from my mind. I remembered that there was a song that we teach to little children naming the books of the bible and I started to sing it to the doctor. The tears started running down my face. I couldn't get past Deuteronomy. How very, very sad. I felt so incredibly stupid. How could I be a pastor, if I couldn't even name the building blocks of my faith? What was wrong with my brain?

Individuals with Alzheimer's disease often experience challenges in memory and recall.

The Diagnosis

I sat in my doctor's office as he looked through all the results of all the tests. He was very caring—and he chose his words carefully. "Cynthia, you need to stop working. You can't do this anymore. You've done an amazing job of trying to hold it together, but it's never going to get better. It's only going to get worse. You've got amnestic mild cognitive impairment and I think it's due to Alzheimer's disease." I'm not sure what else he said after that. I don't remember. But I knew that he was right. That's what was wrong with my brain. I wasn't imagining my memory issues. They were real, just like the MRI's that showed the shrinking of the memory area of the brain called the hippocampus, the thinning of the entorhinal cortex and throw in the fact that I had two copies of the "Alzheimer's gene" (APOE4). Looking back now, my diagnosis really wasn't a huge surprise—a sadness, yes. My mom died of AD and so did her only brother. I was 58 years old.

People with Alzheimer's may have trouble following or joining a conversation. They may stop in the middle of a conversation and have no idea how to continue or they may repeat themselves. They may struggle with vocabulary, have problems finding the right word, or call things by the wrong name (e.g. calling a "watch" a "hand-clock").

Endings & Beginnings

On May 29th, 2011, I stepped into the pulpit for the last time as the Pastor of the Waverly Presbyterian Church. I have no idea how I got through the service other than by the grace of God. The farewell reception was surreal. I walked around the social hall with a box of tissues, sobbing. I was numb. I felt as though I was at my own wake. That week, I started packing up my office and things in my house and I gave away more than 500 books that I could no longer read or reference. Imagine getting a fatal diagnosis, having to leave your job and on top of that, having to move out of your home. It was beyond stressful. I found an apartment in a nearby community (Elmira, NY). The move was tough for many reasons. I felt lonely and scared. It felt as though I was in a bad dream and I just wanted to wake up and find normal again.

FACT: Of the estimated 5.5 million Americans living with Alzheimer's dementia in 2017, an estimated 5.3 million are age 65 and older and approximately 200,000 individuals are under age 65 and have younger-onset Alzheimer's.

From Why Me? to What Next?

There was an ad in the paper for an 8-week class for newly diagnosed individuals, so I signed up and drove to the Big Flats Community Center. My courage evaporated, and I sat in the car crying. When I had no more tears, I got out of the car and started a new chapter in my life. When the classes were over, there was nothing else being offered for those of us with a diagnosis, so I volunteered to help do something—anything to stay busy and find my footing. I wrote the CEO of the Alzheimer's Association in Rochester and was invited to join the Early-Stage Advisory Committee. I offered to reach out to newly diagnosed individuals and to lead a support group. I started feeling useful again. I felt that I had a purpose in life. I started speaking at local service organizations about Alzheimer's disease. I continue to raise funds and advocate for those living with a diagnosis and do what I can to reduce the stigma. I participate in clinical trials. I remember that devastating day in the cemetery and the words of the prophet Jeremiah resonate in my heart: *"For I know the plans I have for you," declares the Lord, "plans to prosper you and not to harm you, plans to give you hope and a future."* Alzheimer's wasn't the end, but the beginning of my new ministry.

Adventures of a Substitute Preacher with Alzheimer's

Rev. Dr. Cynthia Huling Hummel (Presbyterian Church, USA)

On the Road with God

I serve as a substitute preacher for a half dozen or so very small congregations in and around the Finger Lakes in New York—and when I say small, I'm talking about 10–20 folks in worship and that usually includes the organist and myself. It is an exercise in faith, hope and love—for the congregation and for me! **Faith:** that despite my cognitive problems, God will guide us through the worship service and use me to deliver a message. **Hope:** that nothing major goes wrong during the service and **Love:** that I love these little churches and the folks in these churches seem to love me despite my shortcomings and memory lapses.

It Is What it Is

I have always been very open about my Alzheimer's diagnosis. I have done presentations during coffee hour and shared information about resources, programs and services during the announcements. I have also asked for prayers for those living with AD and related dementias, for care partners and researchers. Moreover, I have shared some of the symptoms of Alzheimer's disease, such as forgetting words or getting confused, so folks in these churches wouldn't be alarmed if anything happened to me during a worship service. Moreover, I wanted to give them some ideas on how they could help me if such a situation occurred (and it has). Here are some of the things we have talked about that help me as a substitute preacher living with Alzheimer's disease.

Name Tags

There are some Sundays when I have absolutely no idea who I am speaking with. What can I tell you? It's awkward and crazy-making, especially if they think that I know them. (NOT!) Sometimes I am able to preempt a conversation and ask someone to remind me of their name because I'm having a "memory moment." But many times, it's simply impossible and so I look for ways to end the conversation graciously. More often than not, I am left wondering: who was that person I was chatting with? One of the symptoms of Alzheimer's disease is trouble remembering names and faces. It takes me 6–8 meetings before I can get a new person into my brain's crumbling database. It is very frustrating for me, but I can't hurry the process—it takes eight meetings, period! Moreover, it's got to be more than exchanging names and shaking hands in order for me to learn a new name and face. It means having eight meaningful, face-to-face conversations before anyone new gets added to the ramshackle rolodex in my brain! And here's the kicker: if I don't see that new person for a while, we have to start the process all over again. Yep, eight more meetings! I tell people it is like a game of "Chutes and Ladders." So what's a substitute preacher with dementia to do? I ask folks in the congregations that I serve to PLEASE wear name tags. They usually do it for one Sunday and that's that. I can't begin to tell you how much resistance I get from churches about name tags. "We know who we are. Why do we have to wear name tags?" My answer is simple: "So I can call you by your name." I get so much push back. "Well you know ME!!" Arrgh. It's infuriating. Just because I happen to remember someone's name one day, which trust me, is a miracle, doesn't mean that I will know that person's name the next time I visit the church. Moreover, just because I can read a name on a name tag, doesn't mean that I know or remember anything about that person. That's my reality. It is what it is. Name tags not only help visitors, they help a visiting preacher who is living with Alzheimer's! Name tags also help church members who have cognitive problems to feel more at ease. One of the reasons that folks with dementia drop out of faith communities is because of embarrassment of not remembering names. Dementia-friendly congregations use name tags at all events.

Be Gracious and Helpful

One Sunday, as I was announcing a hymn, a gentleman started waving his hand. "Excuse me, Pastor Cynthia. Do you think now would be a good time to take the offering?" OOPS! I had skipped over it in the bulletin. I said, "Great idea!" I laughed, then everyone laughed and it broke the tension. The ushers then took care of the offering. On another Sunday, I could NOT find the scripture reading for the day. I flipped frantically through the pages of the pulpit bible to no avail. The reading was simply nowhere to be found. As I searched, I wondered if I had a defective bible. I was so mad at myself for not marking the bible reading before the service started. What was the matter with me? Time was ticking and I was flipping back and forth in the Bible and trying not to flip out. I was so busy flipping pages that I didn't notice that a woman from the congregation had walked right up to the pulpit, with an open bible: "Here you go, Pastor Cynthia. The passage is right here. Would you like me to read it for you?" Talk about an answer to prayer. Dementia-friendly congregations practice gracious helping.

Expect the Unexpected and Deal with It

One Easter, I was horrified when I realized that the last page of my sermon was missing. Fortunately, I knew the Easter story well enough and I was able to wrap it up with a line about Mary Magdalene running off to go to tell the others...and then I asked the congregation: "Who will you tell?" Amazing! Like a gymnast, I stuck the ending. Hallelujah! True, the sermon sort of ended abruptly and yes, it was shorter than usual—but hey, I got through it with the help of God's grace. And by the way, the last page of the sermon was safe at home on my printer. I try to keep it all together and remember all the things I need to remember, like showing up at the right church! One thing I know for certain—something WILL go wrong on a Sunday morning. Usually, it's something small like the Sunday that I showed up with the wrong sermon. I had grabbed the wrong one from my file cabinet. Hey, these things happen (at least they seem to happen to me) and while I usually beat myself up over mistakes, I try to remind myself that God might have wanted me to preach the "wrong" sermon because it was the "right" message for someone in the pews that week. One Sunday, I got to church and discovered that I hadn't picked up a sermon at all, but had instead brought a paper that I had written for my class at Elmira College. So during the anthem, I wrote down the three points that I had actually remembered from the sermon that was sitting at home on the dining room table. I shared the points and opened up the sermon inviting the congregation to share their experiences. It was a different sort of sermon—but it wasn't bad. In fact, there was a lot of blessing as folks in the pews, shared their experiences with one another. Sometimes, people will ask me to announce something and I will forget to do it. Sometimes, I will say "trespassers" while the folks in the pews say "debtors." I remind myself, that it is not the end of the world and that I am doing the best I can. A dementia-friendly congregation meets people where they are and celebrates the gifts and talents each one brings—and that includes a substitute preacher with dementia.

When It's Time

There will come a time when I am no longer able to lead worship on Sunday mornings. That's the reality of this disease. The folks in the pews will know that it's time for me to stop, because worship will start to feel uncomfortable. I may say or do inappropriate things or get so lost in the service that people don't know what to do. And so when it's time, I ask for kindness and help in transitioning to a new role. Please help me find other ways to serve. Perhaps I could sing a solo, hand out bulletins, or offer a blessing in worship. Those of us who are living with Alzheimer's or a related dementia are often not the best judges of what we can or can't do, so this news may come as a surprise to me. When it is time for me to "retire" as a substitute preacher, please tell me with love! I don't know how I will react to the news. I may be weepy. I may be relieved. I may be angry or suspicious. I ask now for forgiveness, if I give folks a hard time or say unkind things. Please know that I love you and I have loved preaching in your church and being part of your church family. When I'm no longer able to come to worship with you, please help me to stay connected to God. I love singing the great old hymns of the church. I love the rhythm of the Latin mass and chanting the psalms. I love singing the Shabbat service. I love hearing familiar Bible passages like the 23rd Psalm and praying the Lord's Prayer (with debts/debtors, please!). Even though I may not remember people and events in my life, I believe in my heart of hearts, that I will remember the LOVE and I know with certainty, that the God of Love, will always remember me.

A Prayer on Behalf of Persons Living with Dementia

Dear Lord,

Bless those of us who are living with a diagnosis of Alzheimer's or a related dementia. When days are difficult, wrap us in a blanket of your love and comfort us with your presence and your peace. When nights are dark, give us a star to follow—a nightlight in the heavens to remind us that you are there—guarding and guiding us and lighting our paths. When we are discouraged, give us hope. When we are hopeless, give us faith. When we are weary, carry us close to your heart. When we feel depressed or angry, soothe us. Wipe away our tears and our fears and help us to move from "Why Me?" to "What Next?"

We thank you for our care partners, for our family and friends who are walking with us on this strange and difficult journey. Give us all strength and courage and a sense of purpose as we join our hands and hearts to help others we meet along the way.

Help us all to cultivate an attitude of gratitude each and every day. Remind us to look for blessings in everyday, and holy moments: walking in the rain, singing a familiar song, reminiscing over old photos.

Lord, we pray for the doctors and nurses and all who care about us and for us. We pray for the researchers who are searching for treatments, therapies and cures. Most of all, Lord, we pray for a world without Alzheimer's. Thank you! Amen.

Rocks in My Head

Greg O'Brien (Roman Catholic)

Dr. Seuss once observed, "You've got brains in your head and feet in your shoes. You can steer yourself any direction you choose" (1990).

Not if you have rocks in your head.

My mother always said I had rocks in my head, ever since I was a boy, perhaps the yoke of being an Irish American. Now, decades later, the rocks have calcified, horribly obstructing signals to the brain. Alzheimer's will do that, as it did with my mother, my maternal grandfather, and my paternal uncle. And before my father's passing, he, too, was diagnosed with dementia. Now the demon is coming rock hard for me. Several years ago, I was diagnosed with Early Onset Alzheimer's after a battery of clinical tests and brain scans, and after traumatic head injuries that doctors say unmasked a disease in the making. I also carry the Alzheimer's marker gene, APOE-4.

I've walked in both roles as a caregiver and now as a patient. As the oldest boy in an Irish family of ten, I was the family caregiver on Cape Cod for my parents during their assaults with Alzheimer's and dementia. After my diagnosis and a wallow in a pity party, the Lord pulled me out of my black hole, and exhorted me to get back in the race—the sprint of persistence and endurance for the prize of the old and new testaments. When we are weak, my mother always taught me, God is strong. I've learned the hard way. I have rocks in my head.

For the record, I'm a perfectly, imperfect person, an individual who over time has committed every sin imaginable but murder and adultery, and I've been tested in both. Yet I have been blessed with a gut, unshakeable faith; it is a gift that I embrace more and more with progressions of this disease. Alzheimer's and other forms of dementia, I firmly believe, must be fought on medical, personal, and spiritual realms. I wish I had all the answers; hopefully those reading will glean from first-hand narratives and expressed points of view how faith, hope and humor sustain in dementia. While the mind and body are doomed to fail, the soul survives. In the Lord, one never dies in the strict definition; we just move on to the peace, bliss, and love of eternity—the prize.

With my diagnosis, I turned as a sinner, reluctantly at first, to the one I trust most, God. There was no place else to run. No one understood the disease. How could I expect them? But one must be humbled before being exalted in the Lord. Back to basics, and so there I went.

Over time, I was urged in the Spirit, as spurred in my beliefs, to put on the Mind of Christ, as expressed in the Book of Corinthians. I believe the Lord told me, "Your mind will wither, but my mind will not decay."

I've held to that. It has sustained me. I'm not letting go.

Rocks have held my attention ever since I was a young boy summering on Cape Cod. Leaving the Cape at the end of the season, returning home to Rye, New York outside Manhattan, was always a sad experience for me. I can remember the empty feelings as I filled my duffel bag—the sneakers with the holes in the tips, my jeans with sand in the pockets, a surfing jam bleached by the sun, my wrinkled baseball cap—and carted it out to the station wagon. It always seemed to rain that day.

About a half hour before the family was ready to leave, all 10 of us, I would take one final walk from the cottage off Herring Brook Road in Eastham to nearby Thumpertown Beach on Cape Cod Bay. Along the way, I'd relive the summer—days fishing on Salt Pond, the times we hiked to the Old Coast Guard station, the bicycle rides along the back roads to Orleans, the soothing pounding of the ocean, the sweet smell of beach plums. Each memory was precious as time was slipping away. The memories...

When I reached the crest of the beach, I paused for one last look with the hope that I could freeze the moment in my mind. I then walked down the wooden steps to the beach—each of the 32 planks creaking from summer wear and tear; the gray paint peeling back; many of the nails rusted from the sea air. I could see the charred remains of Labor Day campfires that had blazed the night before. Once on the beach, I ceremoniously walked, as I did each year, to the lip of placid Cape Cod Bay.

There is something ethereal, spiritual, about a Cape Cod summer that, to me at least, no other summer place can match: The sky is brighter, the sun more radiant, the sand softer, the air more pure, the mood more peaceful. The Lord shines here. Like many before me, I sought some tangible connection to this fragile, narrow sliver of land—something, a part of me, which I could leave behind. And so each year at this time, I would walk the beach looking for a special rock, a memory to file deep within. It had to be perfect in every detail—symmetric, polished and about the size of my fist. It had to have just the right feel. It had to feel a part of me.

I usually picked up about three-dozen rocks until I found the right one—my memory of that Cape Cod summer. The rejects were tossed into the bay for more polishing. I then walked back to the staircase and buried my treasure about 12 inches from the foot of the stairs.

All winter long in New York, I'd think of my rock; the summer memories it conjured up helped me through the dreary days.

Then each summer when we returned to the Cape, the first thing I'd do, after unpacking the duffle bag, was to race to the beach to retrieve the rock. I always found it, of course. I had convinced myself—and tried to persuade my mother, the hero of my life—that any rock of similar size was the one I had stored. I collected these rocks in the backyard of the cottage we always rented, walking over them barefoot at times like a cobblestone path to a paradise.

Little did I know at the time that in carrying the rocks back from the beach, ones in the moment that felt the essence of me, I was holding God, not me, in the palm of my hand.

A decade or so later, the Lord was in the palm of my hand, yet again. As a 24-year-old, a cub reporter at The Cape Codder newspaper, I was out of sorts, confused, questioning every belief, every spiritual inkling. Raised Irish Catholic, serving at Mass as an altar boy, Master of Ceremonies to be exact with the designated bishop, I was spoon fed belief; then I rejected it all, turning my back on God and church. I found joy in the moment at a local bar on the Great Outer Beach in neighboring Wellfleet, the Beachcomber. I was no altar boy then, but such temporal bliss can be fleeting in a trek as a young man to question God, the universe, or anyone who would listen. I wanted answers. And so I was drawn early one summer night from the Beachcomber by the magnificence of a remarkable moonless sky with an endless spectrum of stars, as if someone had painted the heavens with flecks of white on an evening when the wraithlike trail of the Milky Way was visible to the naked eye. For a better look, I drove instinctively in my beat up Triumph Tr6, top down, to nearby Four Mile Beach, now called Whitecrest, where I had surfed as a kid. Sitting high on a bluff about 150 feet above the ocean, I sipped in the view, as a spate of questions raced through my head: is God real; who is Jesus; was the universe created by chance; are we just the product of an amoeba; who am I? Damn it, who am I?

I was firing questions like clay pigeons in a skeet shoot, and God, the universe, not sure who at the time, was shooting them down. Pop. Pop.

Pop. No other way to say this, but I was drawn in, felt in the moment that I was in a conversation with someone, not sure who, but began to trust that the heavenly view before me was not created by chance, and that all of us have a purpose. I kept coming back at night throughout the summer. The conversation continued. My trust grew.

Months later, in early September, I went for a run on stunning Nauset Beach in Orleans. With the approach of the Fall Equinox, the sun lowers and the sky turns a perfect azure blue. On this particular afternoon, with a slight wind at my back, I felt a peace I had never experienced. The peace intensified. Finally in my trust, I cried out, "Lord if this is you, let me feel you."

Within seconds, I was sobbing and knelt quietly in the sand. I heard clearly that day in my heart, in my soul: "Yes, I am real, and I will never leave you!"

I've never looked back in doubting God. Though I am ashamed of my walk at times, I know the Lord is real, and will never leave me. There are worst things than sin, I have learned—giving up!

I've held to this faith in my serpentine journey with Alzheimer's—ups, downs, loss of self, self-esteem, judgment, loss of dignity, disintegration of filter, hallucinations, rage, the darkest of isolation, penetrating fears, dramatically reducing one's bandwidth; but, there is great peace in the knowledge that I am not in control any more, and that I am not alone. I've learned over time, through the example of my mother, to write and speak from the heart, place of the soul—one foot here, one in the next realm.

Joseph John Campbell, the renowned American mythologist, writer, and lecturer of the last century, once observed, "We must be willing to let go of the life we've planned, so as to have the life that is waiting for us" (1991).

Irish author C.S. Lewis, Belfast born in 1888 and who came to faith, by his own admission, "kicking, struggling, resentful, and darting his eyes in every direction for a chance to escape," stated in his iconic work, *Mere Christianity* (2015), "Nothing you have not given away will ever really be yours."

And so it is with control. I've learned through my disease that one relinquishes control to gain control at the foot of a higher power. That's the blessing of this disease. Let go, and let God.

Loss of control has relevance on so many fronts with Alzheimer's and other forms of dementia. There is much confusion today over the terms:

Dementia is the umbrella term for cognitive impairment; Alzheimer's is the most prevalent form of it. In all, there are numerous dementias, including vascular dementia, dementia with Lewy Bodies (DLB), Parkinson's Disease, Frontotemporal dementia, Huntington's Disease, and others. The point here is that cognitive impairment, whether it be Alzheimer's or another form of dementia, robs one of self in a desperate search for answers. Often, the progression is gradual, at first outside the view of most others. Finding a handle on losing control can be as challenging and slippery as walking in simple faith. Letting go is most difficult, the reaching out part. That control thing. The irony of dementia is that it can bring us, kicking and screaming, to the essence of yielding imperfectly to a perfect God.

When one surrenders control, instinctively we strive for something in return. The bargaining process. And so in the spiritual, we seek strength and reinforcement from God, and from our ministers, priests, rabbis, Imams, pujaris, Buddhist monks, or other spiritual teachers. But for those on the journey of cognitive decline, we often expect too much from our earthly dons, though they walk in vital roles as critical to us as world-class neurologists and medical experts.

It is difficult to separate the mind from the soul; the mind is the gateway. Many in the spiritual dome don't fully comprehend dementia; like most of us, the word literally scares the hell out of them, a biblical demon howling in the desert, or many perhaps opt for the simple drive by—a smile, handshake, "hi ya," a handoff of a scriptural verse, a reassuring word, or a blank stare—then off to work the flock at large, assuming dementia is a one-size-fits-all disease, akin perhaps to a tent and awning warehouse. Who could blame them. But there is much to learn, much to do, in the spiritual fight against Alzheimer's, poised to take out the Baby Boom Generation and generations to come. The numbers are staggering. Every three seconds, the experts say, someone in the world develops dementia, now ranked the third leading cause of death after heart disease and cancer in the U.S., and is expected to surpass both in years to come. Alzheimer's and other forms of dementia are the only major disease significantly on the rise and for which there is no cure. You can't remove a brain. Today, more than 5.7 million Americans and almost 50 million people worldwide are affected. Experts predict that 150 million worldwide will have Alzheimer's and related dementias by 2050. The cost is equally numbing, affecting family finances and the world at large. The Alzheimer's Association reported in a study entitled, "Changing the Trajectory of Alzheimer's Disease: A National Imperative," that in the absence of disease-modifying treatments, the cumulative costs of care for people with Alzheimer's from 2010 to 2050 will exceed $20 trillion, in today's dollars (2010).

It's been said that there will be two types of people in the world soon: those with dementia, and those caring for someone with dementia. So look around your congregations and places of worship. The scope encompasses just everyone in a seat or standing against a wall, either in the throes of dementia today or heading in the direction as a patient or caregiver.

"We know that Alzheimer's disease is not just 'a little memory loss'—it is a national crisis that grows worse by the day," says Harry Johns, President and CEO of the Alzheimer's Association (Alzheimer's Association 2010).

Notes George Vradenburg, co-founder of the Washington, D.C.-based UsAgainstAlzheimer's, "Alzheimer's is an epic disease. It will take us down...I think it's no question that in fact Alzheimer's will be the financial sinkhole of the 21st century" (personal communication).

To understand Alzheimer's and other forms of dementia, to witness and minister to those with this unspeakable disease, one must first look inside the mind of dementia, understand the disease as best as possible. So what does that look like? Well, not what most people think. This is not your grandfather's disease; it's a family disease.

Alzheimer's is a cunning demon that pilfers a sliver of your brain every day, a death-in-slow motion, robbing one of self, that can take 20 to 25 years to run its serpentine course. And the pathology, experts note, can begin when one is in their 40s. Alzheimer's can also be sexist. Two-thirds of its victims and caregivers are women. In addition, it can be racist. Given statistics, African Americans are 2–3 times as likely and Latinos are 1.5 times more likely to develop Alzheimer's than white Americans. But no one is safe. Alzheimer's respects no demographic, no gender, race or religion. If there ever were a bipartisan issue to stand on, it is for swifter, earlier diagnosis and a cure.

Please don't be fooled by inaccurate stereotypes of this disease; Alzheimer's is just not the end stage when one is unaware of self. There are millions of individuals today living with Alzheimer's in the early stages, sitting in your pews, still highly functioning, perhaps not even diagnosed yet, who are fighting off dreadful symptoms daily, often alone. Those on this journey aren't stupid; we just have a disease that at times, often without notice, takes us down—dramatically diminishing, more and more, our ability to function. Our daily assault against Alzheimer's and other forms of dementia is like the perennial nightmare when one is desperately trying to outrun a monster. While sprinting can work for several laps, slowly the monster overtakes and pounces, as one becomes frozen in time. That's the chilling fear of this journey.

It's been said that Alzheimer's and other forms of dementia are like snowflakes; no two patterns are alike, which greatly complicates the art of ministering. Why are some taken out earlier, while others, like in cancer, fight on longer? If I knew why I could tell you how many angels can dance on the head of a pin. In my case: 60 percent of my short-term memory can now be gone in 30 seconds; I don't recognize people I've known all my life, including my wife on two occasions; I experience penetrating, horrific hallucinations, fly into inexorable rage when the light in the brain goes out; I have a debilitating loss of filter, judgment and time and place. I have no feeling in both my feet up to my knees, and sustain blackouts and right side of body collapsing without notice, given the brain signals have gone awry. And I have cancer that I'm not treating; it is my exit strategy.

Stephen King could not have designed a better plot!

So how does one minister in this disease? In a word: love, the essence of God. But ministering in love to those with dementia and their caregivers, many of whom are at different stages in the disease, requires far more than quotes from scriptures, Torah, Quran, or other readings. It requires the ability to speak to the heart, the place of the soul—the capacity to minister that all is not lost when it appears to be. It requires great discernment.

Given the reality of how dementia affects individuals differently, conventional wisdom on ministering to those in the disease, despite best of intentions, falls somewhere short of reality. Such conventional approaches, to date, are generally geared for those in later stages, arguably only half of the population with dementia, given its long track and earlier stages that can run the course of two decades. From what I've witnessed, advice on ministering to those in later stages of dementia is spot on: creating dementia-friendly places of worship; simplifying services and church activities where possible; offering a greater sense of dignity; incorporation of more music into services; special services and outreaches where possible for those with dementia and their caregivers; ministering to the heart and soul of those with dementia and their caregivers; reinforcement of self-esteem; understanding that those with dementia aren't stupid, we just have a disease; recognizing that our souls aren't afflicted, just our minds.

But what about ministering to those in the early stages of dementia, or those who fear a diagnosis—individuals who are suffering privately and intensely outside the view of others, including their ministers, while working, raising families, trying to pay bills and avoid bankruptcies. What about them? We need ministering, too. To quote the great Bugs Bunny in a classic cartoon, "How about me, boss?" Many of us in dementia battle the symptoms daily like prizefighters. Our heads are bloodied, but unbowed, to borrow from William Earnest Henley in his seminal poem *Invictus*. Sadly, those in later stages may not be as aware of their plights, or rightfully so have taken sabbaticals in life.

But what about us? We're not looking to be overly indulged; we don't want too much hand-holding; we want to be as independent as possible for as long as possible. And we want to be understood. Candidly, it is difficult when one turns to the Lord in dementia for strength, then can't find reinforcement in places of worship because we just don't fit the stereotype of dementia, an observation about as accurate as the sun rising in the west and setting in the east, or those around us engaging in the casual drive-by. "Well, you look so good..."

Bullshit. Excuse my French, but many of those in early or mid stages of dementia are greatly upset, no...really pissed, that we are so misunderstood, that proportionately few really care 'cause we often "look so good." It's almost akin to a deaf person telling an observer: "Do I look like I'm mute?" The takeaway for many in early stages of dementia is that the universe at large seems to only care when someone urinates on the floor in public, soils their pants, or stares blankly into space. Well, many of us are doing that right now outside your views, simply because we still have the capacity to seek privacy. Losing continence happened to me again the other night at the grocery checkout line, and I had to slip out the door with my son, my jeans sopping wet.

Most of us in dementia still want to contribute in so many ways—some spiritual and in other ways. We just need some help, guidance, and encouragement along the way. Dementia, in a twist of ironies, as noted above, can be a blessing of sorts, a gradual loss of control that precipitates an imperfect reach to a perfect God, walking in the reality of our lives, however wrenching. The Lord doesn't cause disease, but finds ultimate victory in it.

Years ago, as a younger man, the perfect sinner who knew better, I was drawn to a verse in the Old Testament, Isaiah 6.8: "Then I heard the voice of the Lord saying, 'Whom shall I send? And who will go for us?' And I said, 'Here am I. Send me!'" (*New International Version*). Instinctively, I prayed it every day, perhaps in an Irish contrition. Be careful what you wish for.

The Lord now has taken me at my word, and I am midcourse, as many of us, between the revelation of sin and the light. "He who has an ear, let him hear," (Revelations 2.7, *English Standard Version*).

The walk in dementia, I've learned, is not just about disease, but the passing into light with grace, a path we all walk in free will. That's the lesson for me, I believe. And so I was asked recently: what are my spiritual needs now; how could clergy best address them; how has prayer changed; what does hope mean; what are the biggest spiritual struggles?

My spiritual need, and the need of so many others in dementia, is to feel loved for our imperfect natures and encouraged to seek our full potentials. This can best be delivered from ministers and congregants who first look within, who come to realize that this walk could be theirs someday, and in many cases likely will.

Hope to me means the prize, an eternal life free of sin, fear and pain—infinity with a loving God; hope means striving to override the mind, speaking from the heart and soul, and embracing challenge.

What are my biggest spiritual struggles? Well, that's another story.

~~~

In his celebrated poem, *Do Not Go Gentle Into That Good Night*, Dylan Thomas urged, "Rage, rage against the dying of the light." (1952). I rage today against the dying light. The distinguished Welsh poet Thomas, with his forceful lyricism and assailing passion, lit a flame in me years ago about the struggle to survive.

Alzheimer's is a dry wick. The spark of the disease that took many of my family members has now ignited me.

Darkness can be a time of greater confusion, anger, and explosive rage in this journey as "sundowning" takes over, a neurological phenomenon of Alzheimer's.[1] I call it the "light switch" effect in the brain: the light is on, the light is off, the light flickers, then goes dark again. This also occurs often when neurons are not connecting properly, and those of us in the disease lash out unexpectedly, often far outside the traits of our personalities—cursing, taking the Lord's name in vain, screaming, hurling insults, even throwing objects without warning, like cellphones, utensils, shoes, and other things, as I have more and more. The rage fuels paranoia like a rocket booster.

1 www.mayoclinic.org/diseases-conditions/alzheimers-disease/expert-answers/sundowning/faq-20058511
~~~

Those of us on this journey are not callous, uncaring, or intentionally unhinged; we just have a disease we can't control. Such behavior can be initiated by loud, throbbing noises, penetrating confusion, excruciating stress, primal fear, cerebral numbness, paranoia, or all of the above.

Profane language can be common in Alzheimer's and other forms of dementia—an expression of gut rage and loss of filter, along with inadvertent grabbing, kicking and pushing, all part of the loss of control in the disease. I don't worry, at this point, that I would hurt anyone; yet I worry that I might hurt myself in moments of overpowering anger, as I've been tempted to do in the past.

I am haunted by the guilt of it. There have been three times that doctors have told me in recent years that I was supposed to be dead: two traumatic head injuries, one from a bicycle accident without a helmet, the other a car crash where my head cracked the windshield, then a time not long ago I intentionally ignored a bleed-out from a prostate cancer biopsy, hoping to end the journey. I didn't tell family or doctors about the excessive bleeding, until the hand of God was upon me. "You don't have the right to do this," I felt in my spirit.

In all, before seeking help, I lost eight pints of blood and was kept at the hospital for three days to be transfused with six pints. Still not getting it, and in deep depression the other night, I entertained stepping off a curb into on-going traffic. The Lord and God's angels pulled me back again, hoisted me out of the black hole. Angels have saved my sorry butt so many times in life!

I believe in angels.

With little left in the tank, I recently went to speak with my pastor about all this and about the incessant rage of this disease, seeking redemption from the shame of on-going, endless invectives. I told my close friend, Rev. Doug Scalise, that at times I hurl profanities at God that would likely raise hairs on the back of Beelzebub's neck. While I've been told the Lord has big shoulders, and embraces straight talk from the heart, I still feel the force of guilt, yet I am humbled by grace.

"We all have a shelf life," Doug tells me, as I reach out for guidance. "We're designed with built-in obsolescence."

Scalise, who earlier faced a life-threatening heart disorder, the "widow maker," as it's called, knows what it's like to walk through the Valley of Death. In fact, he has a copy of the 23rd Psalm in his office: "Though I walk through the valley of the shadow of death, I will fear no evil..."

The verse speaks to all of us.

"You can't helicopter over the valley," he tells me. "You gotta walk through it. Mountain hikers know this. The valley is dark and often you can't see around the next corner; you just have to keep walking."

"Alone?" I ask.

Scalise, a man of considerable wisdom, points to a photo in his office of a flock of high flying geese. With the juxtaposition of the photo, it appears the geese are flying past the moon. While we're all told in life to soar like eagles, he says, geese fly even higher in flock, "V" formation.

"It's a study of teamwork," he adds. "Geese in formation take turns in the lead, breaking the wind; others in the flock draft off the lead, with each bird honking encouragement and benefiting from the bird in front. They all take turns at the front, the hardest role. It's an exercise in leadership. No one is left alone. And so it should be in life."

The pastor undoubtedly knows why I'm here—the evangelical equivalent to a dark confession box.

"What's happening to me, why am I so angry?" I ask.

"You have a right to be angry," he tells me. "It's okay at times to be angry at God. The book of Psalms is filled with such raw emotion, asking the Lord to 'rouse thyself.' We all think God is sleeping at times. 'Wake up, we say, get on with the job!' The anger is understandable, yet misdirected. God doesn't impart disease, but the Lord will use illness to bless."

Weeks later in a sermon, Scalise reinforces the point, telling the congregation it has a choice when walking through the darkest valley. "Don't squander the opportunity," he counsels. "Grow through what you go through," he says, offering a probing parable of a carrot, egg, and coffee beans in boiling water.

"A young woman," he says, "went to her mother and told her how things were so hard for her. She wanted to give up. She was tired of fighting and struggling. It seemed as one problem was solved, another one arose. Her mother took her to the kitchen. She filled three pots with water. In the first, she placed carrots, in the second she placed eggs, and in the last she placed ground coffee beans.

She let them sit and boil without saying a word. After a while she turned off the burners. She fished the carrots out and placed them in a bowl. She pulled the eggs out, and placed them in a bowl. Then she ladled some coffee into a mug. She then asked her daughter: 'What do you see?'

'Carrots, eggs, and coffee,' the daughter replied. Her mother brought her closer, and asked her to feel the carrots. The daughter did, and noted that they were soft. The mother asked her to take an egg and break it.

After pulling off the shell, she observed the hard-boiled egg. Finally, the mother asked her to sip the coffee. The daughter smiled, as she tasted its rich aroma.

Then the daughter asked, 'What's the point?'"

"The mother," adds Scalise, "explained that each of the objects had faced the same adversity, boiling water, but each reacted differently. The carrot went in strong, hard, and unrelenting, but after being subjected to the boiling water, it softened and became weak. The egg had been fragile; its thin outer shell had protected its liquid interior. But, after being through the boiling water, its inside became hardened. The ground coffee beans were unique, however; after they were in the boiling water, they had changed the water.

'Which are you?' the mother asked her daughter. 'When adversity knocks, how do you respond? Are you a carrot, an egg, or a coffee bean?'"

Pastor Scalise looks up.

"Which one are you?" he asks the congregation.

I'm ducking now in the pew, thinking he's speaking straight at me. There is great wisdom in his edifying words about adversity and redemption.

And so for now, I will not go gentle into that good night. I will in faith, and with coffee cup in hand, "rage, rage against the dying of the light."

Even with rocks in my head...

References

Alzheimer's Association (2010) 'Changing the trajectory of Alzheimer's disease: A national imperative.' Retrieved from www.alzheimersreadingroom.com/2010/05/changing-trajectory-of-alzheimers.html on November 02, 2018.

Campbell, J.J. (1991) *The Power of Myth.* New York: Anchor.

Dr. Seuss (1990) *Oh, the Places You'll Go!* London: Penguin Random House.

Lewis, C.S. (2015) *Mere Christianity, Revised and Enlarged Edition.* New York: HarperOne.

Thomas, D. (1952) *In Country Sleep and Other Poems.* New York: New Directions.

Anchor Me

Truthful Loving Kindness (Noahide)

... To each his own. Please remember that this is MY personal story; your own friend or family member may have no trouble remembering and enjoying new spiritual perspectives.

As Persons With Dementia, with progressive loss in our ability to travel and control our own time, our clothing, and our environment, our belief system may become cloudy and inconsequential, or it might become even more crucial to our identity and personal well-being.

My thirst for spiritual relationship began very young and was always a driving influence for my life. At my insistence for prayer and such things, our family found a church and began regular attendance there well before I became a "Christian" at five years old. *Now my spiritual perspectives have changed dramatically, but memories of WHY I myself made those changes are growing dim. Why do I no longer celebrate the special days that my loved ones celebrate? Why do I celebrate "new" special days?* For the past several years I have been forgetting why my spiritual perspective changed (about ten years ago now). Since my husband has never dropped the "Christian" traditions, I suspect that he will get tired of answering my questions for why I decided that we should no longer celebrate with the traditions I remember. ... And asking is rather useless, since even within minutes of his answer I forget the words...and my mind is again asking "WHY?" Now I remember that I will not understand anyway, so I try to avoid asking. It is unspoken but very much on my mind. ... And it makes me uneasy.

Since early childhood I very much enjoyed the family tradition of together tramping thru the forest on Friday after Thanksgiving, searching for the perfect tree, and the sharp scent of pine filling the house as we installed and decorated the tree later in the month. When I dropped the tradition of Christmas tree about ten years ago, I began suspending glass and porcelain ornaments at various places in our home throughout the year, but this last year we again added a very small decorated tree in our house at the holiday—because I cannot remember why I decided not to.

In my childhood and during our children's youth, we spent many happy hours in elaborate decoration of "Easter" eggs. Soon I suspect you will again find me enjoying those activities, because my theological understanding is going backward in time, as well as all my other memories. Most events from the last five to ten years are not well-retained at this stage of my life, and I suspect that time period will go further backwards as my symptoms progress.

So far I have not questioned my "Torah-observant" practice of 7th-Day, probably because I do not see it as restrictive but rather as a weekly celebration. It is simply the tempo of the week—so why NOT celebrate? ((smile))

But internally I am now questioning my other "Torah-observant" practices. I know that eventually they will fall away since my family does not hold those same values...and I accept that as okay when it happens. I do not want to repeatedly wonder why I have restrictions, and don't want my family to try to convince me to continue a practice that I no longer understand WHY I am doing it. I call that "ritual without reality."

What happened?

After more than thirty years of spending over one hour each day for informal language studies from ancient scriptures, I began Systematic Theology study in 2006, using the well-accepted seminary text of Grudem's *Systematic Theology* (1994) (supplemented by an extensive set of free audio classes I found, personally taught by Wayne Grudem). At that point, my un-labeled cognitive symptoms prevented "standard" time expectation for finishing these six courses in various aspects of systematic theology. It took extra time to finish them, but finish I did. However, I ended up feeling more uncertain than when I began; my "foundation" of Bible history did not feel as solid as I had expected it would. So this feeling triggered a larger perspective of study. During 2006 to 2008 more than eight hours each day were spent with intense analysis for textual content in larger perspective of when and where text originated; how, why, by whom, for whom, and in what circumstances it was produced; what influences were at work in its production; and what original oral or written sources may have been used in its composition. (I discovered this wording for "Biblical Criticism" at TheoPedia.com [Ed. note: this domain now for sale] and found it quite accurate to my personal studies.) My selection of source material began with those accepted in seminary-level study, but I gradually realized these were pre-selecting "acceptable" as according to that seminary's perception for message of scriptures. Sources personally "acceptable" as source material began to vary widely and I ended up taking some courses from Yale in the mix along with many others. I ended up doing a huge amount of reading and accepted very few of these "sources" at face value, but in turn questioned the documents these "sources" used as their own source-documents.

I researched and battled out my personal belief statement before I even realized that I was beginning to lose those reasoning abilities. (But of course I lost the belief statement LOL.) *Since I have spent all this time and energy in research and decision, at this stage I strongly object to others confusing me by trying to change my mind with an hour or two of reasoned or emotional arguments. I no longer have ability to understand your arguments ... or to even understand my own rationale for my decisions.* But I have made my decisions and I remember that they were extremely well thought-out. Do not try to proselytize me with whatever YOU believe or don't believe (spiritually and politically); it is of no benefit to either of us, because I no longer have the ability to make those kinds of decisions.

I took lots of notes during those years (none of which I can now understand), and was devastated at my conclusions. Dropped membership in local "Christian" church, and I cried myself to sleep almost every night for two years, at the dis-illusion of my "Christian" Biblical foundation. Many persons become bitter with these discoveries, but my *relationship* with Creator remained firm.

After those years of extra-intense study my theological stance changed dramatically; on my 50th birthday I changed my legal name to Truthful Loving Kindness (based on Hebrew term "chesed v' emet"), began Torah-observant practices late 2008 and on 27 April, 2011, I formally requested conversion in a rather progressive-minded Jewish congregation while continuing personal study on the origin of Hebrew language. My conversion request was denied, but my conclusions continued to evolve for the next year or two and I continued worshiping with them from 2008 thru 2014. But now I remember meaning for very few of the Hebrew words in the songs or scriptures. The tunes and rituals are vaguely familiar, but do not have the visceral connection of my own childhood traditions... and the newer connections are dropping out. (I give dates above in order to provide context for symptoms.)

I suspect that, as my symptoms continue to develop, I will especially *need* those childhood hymns to keep myself grounded, so I guess it is a good thing my request was denied because I am again in search of a congregation...while I can still be involved in decision-making process. Meanwhile I plan to invite a few friends every week to just sing songs; everything from first two verses of "How Great Thou Art" to "What a

Beautiful World"...or whatever anyone wants to sing. We will open our mouths for sound to come out ((smile)).

I remember much of the vocabulary for what I do believe (and what I disagree with), but no longer remember any of the reasons for agreeing or disagreeing with specific doctrines of organized religion. ... And yet I need to have local persons in like-minded (monotheistic) worship. Long-distance, internet-based connections do not meet the need for voices raised together in song, or a gentle touch on the shoulder. My needs are changing.

Since my dementia symptoms continue to advance, it is definitely a time to reach for those common worship traditions which I will probably need in the future. I pray to find a local congregation soon. ...or maybe we will just continue to sing songs ((smile)).

Note: This submission began as two blog entries at www.truthfulkindness.com, and I have a separate "spiritual" blog at https://tlk4spiritual.wordpress.com.

Anchor Me

Maybe I am drifting,... or maybe connecting and connected to a great mass.
I don't know.

Maybe...
instead of a being of objectivity
...analyzing what I observe,
I am somehow becoming intimately connected with it.

... No longer the observer
but instead a tiny part
of what OTHERS observe and quantify and analyze.

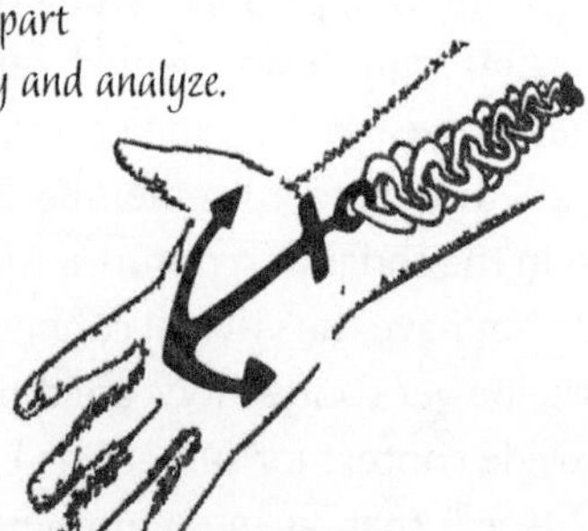

... Maybe I am not going away from life
but instead I am BECOMING life.

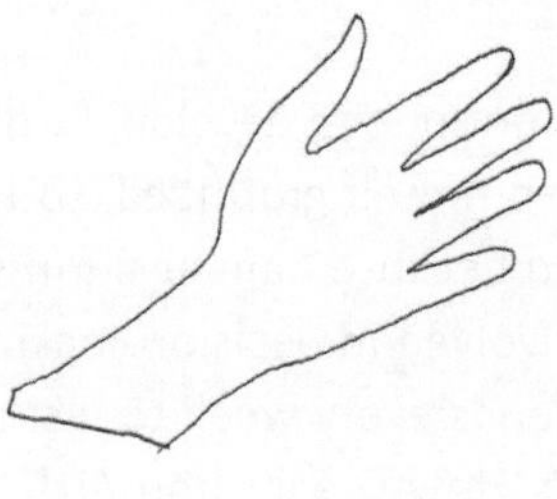

...
But I would like to spend a moment
connected to you instead,
so please hold my hand and anchor me.

...Please.

Truthful Loving Kindness 2012/09/13

Tru here. Always an analyst, this was written very early in my efforts to occasionally step away and observe my own dementia symptoms. ...confused by the new intense non-word connections with something greater, and, at the same time the new distance between myself and most of the persons and tasks in my life. ...adrift.

Wake-up Songs: Be Still My Soul

Jan 07, 2017

Creator values me, and considers me important in the whole scheme of things.

... Just like YOU are, my friend.

Tru here.

This morning I awoke hearing a melody in my head. Like the last time I woke to this tune, almost 10 years ago in late 2007, could not remember any words that went with the melody I was hearing.

Last time I heard this song as a wake-up melody, I sang Mom the tune that woke me. Someone in the room with her recognized that I was humming "Be Still My Soul."[2] *They sang the lyrics for me:*

Be still, my soul; the Lord is on thy side;
Bear patiently the cross of grief or pain;
Leave to thy God to order and provide;
In every change He faithful will remain.
Be still, my soul; thy best, thy heavenly, Friend
Through thorny ways leads to a joyful end.

Be still, my soul; thy God doth undertake
To guide the future as He has the past.
Thy hope, thy confidence, let nothing shake;
All now mysterious shall be bright at last.
Be still, my soul; the waves and winds still know
His voice who ruled them while He dwelt below.

2 Video link: https://youtu.be/duGBIPEusks

Be still, my soul; the hour is hastening on
When we shall be forever with the Lord,
When disappointment, grief, and fear are gone,
Sorrow forgot, love's purest joys restored.
Be still, my soul; when change and tears are past,
All safe and blessed we shall meet at last.

(Catharina von Schlegel, 1697–?; translated by Jane Borthwick, 1813–1897)

My first wake-up song was very early; 4am on April 2, 2006. I thanked God for adding a song to his wonderful alarm clock for prayer time. Two days later, I awoke even earlier (3am) hearing a different song. It would not have surprised me that much if it was a song recently heard. A song is always running thru my head, usually whatever song I heard last. If I do not have focus on something then I am humming it. (Got in trouble from plenty of teachers and employers due to that personality glitch.) So maybe I have just started triggering music at odd times. But my wake-up song was almost always something I had not heard for years; and usually either a hymn or a love song. My default song is "Who Will Buy?" ("...this wonderful morning" from the musical "Oliver") and it is really odd to hear a song in my brain when I have not heard the song from outside my brain first.

During that year (2006–2007) I woke very early morning at least every other day, with a song playing in my head. I would quietly get out of bed, trying not to wake my husband, figure out what song I was hearing, and write as much as I remembered of the lyrics. Almost always they were either an answer to a question I had asked in prayer, or they prepared me for the near future.

But within a few months, many of the songs sounded like I had some very negative changes coming up. I started getting scared ... and I mean it got to where it REALLY scared me. June 13th I heard "Blue Shadows on the Trail," which I had not heard since childhood. Then June 14th I had "Empty Saddles in the Old Corral." I spoke to my Pastor, because with my past experience of dreams and premonitions that came true, this was really scaring me.

"How do I tell what is a message from God, and what is from my subconscious mind? Looking back, it APPEARS that God has 'spoken' through dreams, feelings, and words (as well as, of course, scripture). I had thought my wake-up songs were from Him, but are they really?"

Pastor said he did not have much experience with things like this that really came to pass, but sent me to a couple other folk. Also he reassured me that, with my increasing dis-Abilities, he did not really think these songs forecasting hardship and change meant terrible things for my loved ones, but was possibly just saying to prepare for more intensively difficult times for myself. "Empty saddles includes not only those who are dead—but simply those who are no longer able to ride."

One of my most emotional wake-up songs was 5:30 on June 22, 2006, when I woke to the phrase: "Love me; that's all I ask of you" from Phantom of the Opera. Most of the songs gave instructions to love, rest, or count blessings, but an amazing amount of songs had the instructions to "SING !!!" The others spoke to preparing for hardship.

We now theorize I had my first tiny stroke February 1999. I had become both cognitively and physically dis-Abled by the year 2000, but it all began in 1976, and even tho I spent months with some of the top specialists, doctors were never able to figure out the root of my many problems. I began using a wheelchair during the year 2000, and my dis-Abilities were still increasing in 2006.

Wake-up songs continued thru 2006 and into 2007.

During 2007, we figured out it was a combination of several tick-borne diseases, including both Lyme and Babesia. I began an intensive treatment regime which resulted in my writing that I couldn't eat, sleep, or do anything except huddle, shaking, in a fetal position on the couch.

At 1:15 am on Sept 22, 2007, my wake-up was "... because I love you, just the way you look tonight." I wrote in my journal, "what a forgotten, wonderful song."

I quit writing down the songs on Sept 24, 2007. "If these are from God, then why does no one else get wake-up songs?" I was seriously questioning the source of the songs, and that phase of my life trickled to a close. Now I get a wake-up song once in a while, but not often.

It has been months, or maybe even a year since I have had a wake-up song, and with my dementia symptoms "Be Still My Soul" is oh so very apropos, especially on my second day of being unsupervised and my dementia symptoms reflect an increase from stress. (I was too sick to go with husband for several days of visiting my adult children, and picking up various purchases that had been ordered for pick-up along the driving route.)

I would still love confirmation, but highly suspect these songs are Creator giving me an early-morning hug ... and this morning I needed one ((smile)). Some people get that affirmative hug from an absolutely unique albino bird visiting their back yard, or other unique experiences that "speak" to their particular soul. Mine is a wake-up song ((smile)).

Creator values me, and considers me important in the whole scheme of things.

... Just like YOU are, my friend.

Wake-up Songs: Come Near!

Apr 12, 2017

Tru here. Have not had another wake-up song in past three months, but usually they are just musical phrases of melody playing in my head, with no words. This morning however, there WERE words ... this time with no melody; "Non Dimenticar."[3]

Mom and Dad had this song on a Jerry Vale record when I was growing up, and it has probably been 30 years since I've heard it. So it's been years since I have even thought of this song, but today I woke hearing the words to "Non Dimenticar" in my head. Began this blog entry 6 am on Palm Sunday ... and this year it is the day before Passover begins.

Dementia: the root verb of this phrase, "non dimenticar" [Ed. note: "non dimenticar" means "do not forget"] and a very large issue in my personal life. Along with the strong reminder of Creator's love, this song brings the question: in my time and efforts for dementia advocacy, have I been forgetting to "come near" for intimate time with my creator?

Come near!!

"Draw near to God and He will draw near to you." (James 4.8a, New King James Version)

Command to "come near" is important in my life. About 15 years ago I dedicated almost an entire year to language and context study of the scriptural imperative to "come near." For more than five hours every day, I studied those words in original languages, each scriptural use in context, accessed online articles, and bought some books to check out professional opinions. Then one day my old newfoundland Service Dog, Hero (my first "Hero") was hurting and whining for me to come sit with him. He was asking me to drop everything

3 Here is a video of Non Dimenticar: https://www.youtube.com/watch?v=PkH-KQgDokA

and come close; just sit with him as a fellow being. No touching and no words; just decision to spend time together. So I did. Then (like a light coming on) I realized what "come near" was all about.

The command "come near" is all about human volition; decision to stop the world for spending time with Creator. ... and then DOING it.

After I learned to "come near," Creator and I had some intensely intimate bonding time. This bonding time has created the foundation and context for how I personally handle life with progressive dementia issues.

There is no sharing physical "touch" with a being who has no physical form, but there can be spiritual touch much more satisfying and intimate than holding hands or kissing. And there can be communication without even the need for words in any form. It is as much a "different" format of communication as body language is from written language. Humanity might call it "primitive" because this communication has nothing we recognize as words, but it is even more richly nuanced ... along with being profoundly intimate. It can also be amazingly intense, with results that vary from exhaustion to complete relaxation or invigoration.

Now I need to go, because Creator is waiting for me. (... and waiting for YOU too!)

Creator's love is the anchoring absolute for my life. It is the lodestar of truth which anchors the circumstances in which I find myself, and guides my decisions. Again, I need to go now, because Creator is waiting for me. (... and waiting for YOU too!)

Reference

Grudem, W. (1994) *Systematic Theology.* Nashville, TN: Zondervan.

Me Fe Nos Sostiene (My Faith Sustains Us)

Daisy Duarte (Nondenominational Christian), as told to Lynda Everman and Don Wendorf

---

I say that my faith sustains "us" instead of "me" because I am now taking care of my Mom who has advanced Alzheimer's disease. Her life-long deep faith sustained our family in my childhood, through all kinds of hardships, and the faith she taught me has sustained me through my adult years. Now that she can no longer talk or pray or sing the Christian songs she loves or go to church, my faith that I share with her and for her still keeps us both going and living our passion for the Word of the Lord.

Mom raised my brother and sister and me in the suburbs of Chicago, mostly by herself and in spite of several tough, even abusive relationships. I was the "troublemaker" kid who really gave her a run for her money. Mom got up at 4:00 each morning and rode four buses and one train to work in the inner city as a teacher's aide, regardless of the sometimes harsh Chicago weather. These were often difficult times, but she taught us to have faith: "Dios prevalecerá, tu saldrás bien." "God will prevail; you'll come out of it." It may take years, she said, but you will. She said that "God died on the cross for us and it doesn't matter what we do in life, He's there for us." She made it clear we had to fight our own battles and be independent, but that we could make it by always "seeking God because He's the one who's always there, 24-7." She showed us that "...the same kind of respect you want to get, you have to give to others" and she lived by that idea.

Mom was a devout church-goer and she taught us to love the church. We were baptized as Catholics, although Mom eventually found a nondenominational Bible church that seemed best for her. She went to church every Wednesday and Friday nights and again on Sunday and even found time to cook on Saturdays for homeless people. She appreciated the practical life lessons she heard at church and felt the Lord was "speaking right to her." And we both loved the Christian music and still do.

My brother left for the Marines at about age 17 and when my sister was about 17, she had a baby and moved to Missouri. Mom and I stayed in

Chicago for a time and then I moved to Missouri to work in my sister's and brother-in-law's restaurant. When I was in my early 30s, I opened my own sports bar which I loved doing. But, when Mom was about 55 years old, she started getting sick and showing lots of problems with memory and emotions. She would eventually be diagnosed with Alzheimer's disease when she was 57. We moved Mom to Missouri and I became Mom's caregiver in my home.

I never questioned becoming Mom's caregiver, even when it cost me a romantic relationship when my partner at that time insisted Mom needed to be put in a home. But my faith and the values of the Hispanic community of taking care of our parents ourselves at home made my decision very clear. They did it for us; we have to do it for them. Mom taught us to be independent and to be fighters. My love for her and the help of the Lord keep me going. The only two people I can thank my whole life from the bottom of my heart are my Mom and the Lord.

Mom was misdiagnosed at first and we had some very tough times. For awhile, she was able to help some at my sports bar, but at one point she told my then 13-year-old nephew to stab her with one of the kitchen knives, even though she had seemed her usual happy, social self. I closed the sports bar and took her home, where the next morning she was still crying and screaming, "God, stop telling me to kill myself." She was hallucinating and I took her to the hospital, where they stopped all her medications, which actually helped a little. After a lot more testing they decided she had Creutzfeldt-Jakob disease and would die within six to nine months. I took her home, intending to take care of her there until she died. I promised Mom I would never put her in an institution. That was eight years ago.

I did a lot of research and new doctors and testing finally came up with the diagnosis of Alzheimer's disease. I had had to close down my business and for the next three years I was her full-time caregiver at home. I didn't have any social life and had some depression but was glad she and I could share a lot together, including Christian music we both loved so much. Mom likes the Spanish contemporary Christian music I get on Pandora while I keep my contemporary Christian praise music going all day on my earphones. It keeps us going.

We now have a routine to keep feeding our passion for the Word of the Lord. Mom can no longer go to the New Life Church in Springfield, so we now watch it online together. They have about 60–90 minutes of contemporary Christian worship music and talks on themes like forgiveness, generosity, current social issues, and the real life struggles people go through. I like the practical help. Mom really likes the music which I turn up real loud for her hearing problems. She can't sing anymore but she tries to grunt along on the songs she knows and I sing along with the others for her. Sometimes this really touches me a lot.

Every morning I start our day by kissing Mom and putting my hand on her head as I make the Sign of the Cross on her forehead with my thumb. I pray for us by saying "Thank you Lord for giving us another day of life" and "Thank you for dying on the cross for our sins. Forgive us for any of our sins and may you guide us through our day." Then we do the morning routine of changing diapers, getting cleaned up, feeding her breakfast, getting dressed, combing her hair, and brushing her tongue. On days I work she is taken care of by my nephew and my partner, who put her to bed days I work late at my brother-in-law's restaurant.

Even if she is asleep when I get home, we end the day with the Sign of the Cross again and a talking prayer about how the day went. Then I pray for us and thank God for another day and for guiding us through it. I add that "Whenever you need to give Mom her wings, I know she's ready" if that is His will. I say, "If she's in any pain, let your blood run through her veins and take away the pain."

We also have spiritual help from our congregation. They pray all the time that she be pain free and for the Lord to "give her her wings" as He wills it. The more people are praying for us, the more blessings. God knows how to sort out our prayers. He does what He does and we just have to do what we do. The chaplain from Hospice also comes once a month to give us support and he prays for Mom and for me, which helps a lot.

In the process of finding the right diagnosis for Mom, I learned from her family in Puerto Rico, just how many other family members had had Alzheimer's. It's about 75 percent on my Mom's side, going back for generations. I enrolled in the Dominantly Inherited Alzheimer's Network research study at the Washington University School of Medicine in St. Louis and learned in 2015 that I tested positive for the early-onset familial Alzheimer's gene that is all over my Mom's family. That means that I will probably have the disease by my 65th birthday. I am now in my early 40s, living with the knowledge that my memories have a limited shelf life, set to expire in 25 years. This was all gut-wrenching to go through and I cried when I first heard my diagnosis. But, I want to be able to help my Mom and the rest of the family and the community.

I decided to use my time to fight for a cure as an advocate, a caregiver and as one of the few Latina participants in an Alzheimer's clinical trial. Latinos are 1.5 times more at risk for Alzheimer's and more than 1.8 million Latino family members care for an individual with dementia. Most are daughters like me who believe in taking care of our loved ones ourselves. I also became a spokesperson for LatinosAgainstAlzheimer's and I lobby for Congress to give more funds for research.

Caregiving is a high-stress, around-the-clock job. Often the ones we care for don't remember who we are and cannot dress, feed or bathe themselves. It takes love, a sense of duty and honor, and lots of help from others. But, my Mom taught me: "Si tienes amor sin condiciones, tú puedes emprender todo." "If you have unconditional love, you can tackle anything." She always told us: "Dios prevalecerá, tu saldrás bien." "God will prevail; you'll come out of it." I believe in my Mom and in the Word of the Lord. My faith sustains us.

Be Not Afraid

Jim Gulley (Roman Catholic)

Be not afraid. I go before you always. (John 6.20; *New American Bible*)

When I grew up, September and going back to school were always very special, particularly when I was enrolled in a seminary program in the beautiful Finger Lakes Region of New York State. It was at the southern tip of Seneca Lake, and the school building was a treasured complex, over 100 years old when I lived there, formerly called Cook Academy. The village of Montour Falls was surrounded by magnificent waterfalls and glens. September was the time when the many trees shined in magnificent arrays of color. We knew that this meant that change was beginning to happen. Soon the beautiful outdoors would go to sleep for what seemed like a very long time, but the beauty would re-emerge in the spring following a few short, but difficult months.

September 2004 was the month when I last had a coherent conversation with my dad, also named Jim. As I am now, he was then struggling with Alzheimer's disease. He had a stroke soon after that, was very ill, mostly non-conversant, in a great deal of pain, and in the last stage of Alzheimer's. He might have known us when we visited, but he couldn't acknowledge it. Mostly he watched the world, not having a chance to participate in it any longer. Dad died in July 2005, after spending his last days in the hospital in which he was born. The whole family was there with him for those days, praying for him, trying to comfort him, but without knowing what, if anything he could sense.

Dad had a very humble upbringing in rural Tennessee, much of it during the Depression which hit the South very hard. His parents worked menial jobs including work as sharecroppers. Their family got very low pay, little formal education or medical care. Dad learned self-sufficiency from his parents, along with how to live with hardship with a simplicity of life, tenacity, courage, and belief in fundamental values of faith in God, family love, humility, generosity, and a determination to see the next generation do better. Mom worked as a hospital nurse from when I was born and together, they made just enough to support our family of six kids and to put us through school and college.

As he aged, Dad became more limited in what he could do, and began to manifest signs of dementia. Despite his limitations, I learned from him, confided in him, listened to him. He told me how he feared nursing homes, not knowing that he would live in one for many months. In our last good conversation, I shared with him some of the difficulties of my life. He smiled in his impish Irish way, and told me, "Don't worry, it's okay." He told me he was okay with what was happening to him, and that I should be okay with my difficulties too.

I didn't know it at the time but he was echoing the very comforting words of Isaiah 41 of Hebrew Scripture, John 6.20 of Christian Scripture, and the words written by Prophet Muhammed in the Quran, "Be not sad or afraid, Allah is with us." God told Abram in Genesis 15: "Do not be afraid" because God promised to be his shield and give him a great reward.

Dad's faith was quiet, humble, subdued, strong and constant. Like me, he went away from the church for a while but came back to celebrate life, hope, and community later in life. He became very active in the work of the Knights of Columbus, and his community benefited in important ways from his contributions of time and talent.

Mom's deeply rooted faith was not only critical to her throughout her life, but she set a very visible example to all of us in the family about how to live a joy filled life. Mom's funeral in 2017 was one of the most traumatic and most beautiful experiences I have ever had. I only hope that I can live and die with courage, grace, hope in eternal life, and longing to be with God, as she did.

I had begun to question my own health in September 2015. I was still working, driving, and doing the things that a person of my age would do. But I knew that things would soon be different. I had survived a stroke and heart surgery. It impelled me to focus not only on what changes I was experiencing but also how my life was beginning to mirror my dad's. I was diagnosed with early stage Alzheimer's disease in November 2015. It really didn't take a rocket scientist to predict that this would happen, given the stroke, other symptoms, family history, and initial neurological testing. *(Wait a minute...I once WAS a rocket scientist working at Goddard Space Flight Center in telemetry processing!)*

But I was determined not to take Dad's quiet, isolated life path. Once I met with the neurologist and got the Alzheimer's diagnosis, I was resolute in my commitment to be as open as possible with those I knew, and even those I was meeting for the first time, letting them know that I had been diagnosed with Alzheimer's, even though the symptoms visible to them seemed mild. I knew that this was a serious turn in my life and that my health would only worsen over time.

I was not mad at God. Things just happen. I announced the news of my diagnosis in a parish staff meeting at St. Joseph's Catholic Church and let everyone know that I would continue my work as a Pastoral Associate, visiting those in hospitals, hospices, and in their homes who needed pastoral care and support. I would continue to be active not only in weekend liturgies, but also in the several other church activities that were already important to me: helping prospective new members, leading Scripture study groups, participating in the Knights of Columbus, playing in the hand bell choir, extending outreach to homeless people, helping to feed those in downtown shelters, and other activities, for as long as I could.

My wife Rose and I immersed ourselves in the work of the Rochester and Finger Lakes Chapter of the Alzheimer's Association. We participated in an eight-week "Orientation to Alzheimer's" support group, got involved in the two major fundraising activities in our region: *The Longest Day* and the *Walk to End Alzheimer's*. We participated in an advocacy day at our state capital where we talked to legislators about our personal encounters with dementia and what we needed from them in terms of funding, public visibility, and general awareness. I was named to the National Early Stage Advisory Group based in Chicago. We meet in person twice a year, and then via video conferencing monthly. Many of our dementia peers rely heavily on email, Facebook, chat boards, and conferencing to communicate with each other and with others in our unique dementia "club." Our grown kids, Jen and Dave, have been amazingly supportive and compassionate throughout this ordeal.

About a year ago, I sensed that my symptoms were beginning to intensify. Speech became more problematic. My balance was not as good as before, and I became more prone to falling. Multi-tasking became more difficult, and in a church of over 5,000 members, that was a problem. So I talked with my pastor and made the decision to retire from work as a paid staff member, but offered to continue to perform as many of the same functions as I could, as long as I could, on a volunteer basis. On the last weekend of employment at church, I spoke to the congregation at each service. I told them about the disease, what I expected in the future, and how much more I needed them now, and I asked for their prayers. That day, and every weekend since, dozens of people go out of their way to talk to me, see how I'm doing, and give me a big hug. Hugs are good.

You've heard the term "caregiver." The Alzheimer's Association offers the alternative term "care partner." Caring for an individual with dementia is a life changing experience, for both people in this equation. The caregiver's life is impacted in significant ways, including mental and physical stress, frustration, anger, and the desire to wave a magic wand over the situation. As much as the "care receiver" needs spiritual care, even when their verbal skills fail them, the "caregiver" needs as much or more weekly contact and support from clergy, lay ministers, and other members of the congregation. Both need to receive appropriate medical, mental, and spiritual care in order for this to be an effective partnership. I am blessed to have been married to Rose for nearly 50 years, and to have had her as a care partner for more than two years. She participates in virtually all of our Alzheimer's Association activities, including conferences specifically meant for caregivers. She helps me by identifying coping mechanisms to keep both of us safe. She provides encouragement, sits in on all my doctor's appointments to remember what I forget, and she's at church every weekend ready to provide pastoral care.

I have probably not been this busy in a long time, and I love it. I have done radio interviews, webinars, several speaking engagements, making phone calls for the Association, and writing.

I think the phrase *"Be Not Afraid"* is vitally important for those of us with Alzheimer's and other forms of dementia. It helps so much if we can accept the cards we have been dealt, even though at times, perhaps even over years, it will be a very difficult journey. At times we will think that we have totally lost our dignity, our purpose in life, all ties to our family and friends. Depression is common at times like these. We may want to be alone, to be away from the rest of the world. For many of us, the initial diagnosis was more than we could handle. It caused us to retreat and check out of active family and public life, not always because of physical symptoms, but often because of our fear, self-inflicted embarrassment and changes in our life status. We were once the care *givers*, the sustainers, the source of income, but now we are the *receivers*, sustained by our kids, our spouse or partner, or perhaps even someone we don't know. I've seen it, know it's true, and believe that at some point, it could impact me in the same way. But there are things that we and our caregivers can do about this.

I spoke to my pastor, Father James Schwartz (also a great friend, preacher and counselor) a few days ago, and he reminded me, "Don't let fear hold you back, or any of us back." Those in many faith communities have a firm, unswerving belief in eternal life after human death in communion with God and those from all time in the Church of God. The messages of Scripture and the words of weekend liturgy are critical to faith. So is the ministry of the ordained and lay church ministers to people like me, who are living in the middle to later stages of dementia. Do not try to soft-pedal this disease, telling us we'll be fine. Many of us believe in the credibility of the time worn adage: "God will not give us more than we can handle." Check out the Hebrew Scripture Book of Job. Everything is *not* fine. We need other messages of consolation. Words about the never ending, never failing love of God in return for our love of God. Please don't preach at us with hyper-theological treatises and obscure parable phrases. Instead, please comfort and reassure us. Remind us that God is always ready for a loving, comforting relationship with us, despite our physical and moral frailties.

"Be not afraid" pertains not only to those of us with a dementia diagnosis, but perhaps more so to our spouses, partners, family members and close friends. They become very protective of us; they themselves may become very depressed; and they are often very angry at the loss or loss of control of their lives at the expense of caring for us.

There are many ways pastors and parishioners can be helpful to persons living with dementia and their families. Education is key. The number of people today with this disease is staggering and that number will only increase.

Most of us don't know how to communicate with, or empathize with, persons who have cognitive impairments. If it appears that we don't understand, some people will raise their voices to a point near a shout, and then get flustered and retreat. The problem is not with our ears; it's with our brains! Be patient. If something isn't working, don't be afraid to try another method: perhaps writing on a tablet or showing us something in a hymnal or bible, a bulletin, a newspaper, a book, or even a magazine.

Rather than preach at us, my observation is that effective chaplains and clergy listen carefully. They actively listen, asking to clarify a point, but not quickly responding directly to it. They listen for cues that something is amiss.

We fear what we don't understand. Creating opportunities for those of different faiths to interact can reveal that behind the doctrines of these faiths, we find many similarities. For example, the Golden Rule ("Treat others as you would like to be treated") is found in every one of the world's religions. This shared insight from each of the five largest religions—Judaism, Hinduism, Buddhism, Islam and Christianity—might have meaning to a person with dementia even when you aren't familiar with their particular beliefs and church affiliation.

Sometimes people approach us, and learning of our impairment, express sorrow, even shedding tears. But, we haven't died...at least not yet! Yes, we understand that currently there is no cure or reversal for dementia diseases. But we're getting by. What we need is simply your presence—show up, include us, visit us at home or in a facility, give a hug, offer a smile. We're okay. And we want you to be okay, too.

It may help people inexperienced with dementia to talk with someone who has "gone public" with their diagnosis and is willing to discuss the disease process, either in a personal conversation or in public. There are also many books now written by people living with dementia in which they educate you about the issues and how to address them.

Learn the facts. Those with dementia constitute a big, diverse community of women and men, with ethnic roots from all countries and races, different life stories, situations and needs. Women are twice as likely to have dementia as men and African Americans and Latinos are proportionately more likely than non-Hispanic whites. Up to 5 percent of the more than five million Americans diagnosed with Alzheimer's have early-onset Alzheimer's and are diagnosed in their 40s and 50s: approximately 200,000 people.

Please advocate in every venue possible, not just in a political forum, for better and equal care for dementia treatment for everyone. You can do much from the pulpit, in newsletters and bulletins, and by hosting periodic "non-stigma" retreats or receptions for those in the community who either have a diagnosis, or want to learn more about these conditions. The local Alzheimer's Association, Area Agencies on Aging and other organizations will gladly help with speakers and participate in these events.

Consider periodic worship liturgies in which well memorized hymns are sung and where a shorter, simpler liturgy is used. You might get a higher level of participation from those who are struggling with memory loss and are confused by complex tasks. Cite a simple but powerful phrase of encouragement, peace and comfort from scripture, such as "Be not afraid. God/Allah is with you."

Encourage the choir director to reach out to us with music. Music has been shown to be amazingly effective with many serious diseases, including the dementias.

Encourage lay members to lend a listening ear, a compassionate heart, a smile, and a welcoming attitude, especially those who have formal training in pastoral care.

Offer to drive someone with the diagnosis to church or fellowship activities occasionally to give the caregiver a break, or a chance to worship quietly in their own ways.

Invite local Alzheimer's Association and medical center researchers to meet with your staff and congregation to discuss available resources, opportunities to participate in clinical trials, upcoming events and activities for those of us with Alzheimer's and other forms of dementia.

Work with the local Alzheimer's Association Chapter and other organizations to host a support group in your house of worship, or publish information about who to contact about participating in nearby support groups which match our particular needs.

There are many differences and dimensions to those of us with a diagnosis of Alzheimer's disease, Lewy Body Dementia, Frontotemporal Dementia or other forms of dementia, at so many different levels of invasion and impact. For example, we're not all *old*, although our actions and activities might seem to suggest that. It is unreasonable to approach us all in the same manner, to minister to us in the same way, or to expect us to respond in the same way. Having a stock ministry method for all of us would be a waste of everyone's time. We need to be treated as individuals because we are.

When I spoke to Father James Schwartz, he told me that the most effective way to find out someone's unique situation is simply to ask them. He suggested that ministers should ask "How do you feel being in church with this disease?" Ask open-ended questions. Let the person with the diagnosis take the dialogue where it might go. He advised that a regular conversation should be established early on, especially with those in early and mid-stage dementia, to keep us sharing with our clergy how we are doing and what we need.

Keep sermons brief and to the point. I have had four years of seminary training, four years in a Jesuit College, and three years earning my Masters degree in Theology and Pastoral Care. But each weekend, when I'm in the pew and the preacher approaches the lectern, I hold my breath for a moment wondering what kind of sermon it will be. Will it really be an unwrapping of the day's main Scripture reading? Will it provide a way for me to internalize the good news of the Gospel, given that my cognition isn't what it once was? Will it provide practical suggestions and ideas for how

I can live out the Scripture passage in the week ahead? Or will it be more akin to a theological treatise, a catechetical lecture on leading our moral life? I believe that, from the eyes of one with cataracts in the front of my head, and tau tangles inside my head, that the 1st approach is much more likely to continue my worship during each week. Even with my education background, I am often baffled by the 2nd type of preacher's exhortation which leaves me spiritually unenergized at the end of the liturgy.

One valuable way in which we can get a handle on this is by recalling the teaching of the 20th century theologian, (Jesuit) Father Karl Rahner who taught that the whole of creation is filled with and sustained in the mystery of God's love. The idea that God is only found in religious practices and comes to us solely in church, profoundly misses the mark when it comes to understanding the truth of the Scripture message. According to Rahner, God's gracious presence and loving mercy toward us are not consequences of our celebration of the liturgy in a church building at a specific time. Rahner invited us to live a "Liturgy of the World" in which we demonstrate our faith not only through structured prayers and rubrics, but by being one with all in God's church anytime, anywhere. The Liturgy of the World is God's gift of self to humanity at all times and places. We continue to worship in the most human way when we reach out during the week to those who need our help, including to those of us with dementia, our families, our caregivers. This is a message that we with the diagnosis need to hear.

Some of us with a dementia diagnosis are still able and eager to provide pastoral care and encouragement to others also in our unique, but seldom understood company of those afflicted with dementia (now over 5.7 million in the United States). Congregations need to explore ways to help us continue to contribute and serve.

Encourage those with dementia in your place of worship. Read to those who are no longer able to do this, from Scripture, the Quran, spiritual books. Play an appropriate religious video or sacred music to provide musical uplift during an otherwise depressing day. Very importantly, provide company, consolation, prayer, understanding, and support for us and for those in our families, neighborhood, and broader friendship rings.

Include us in worship roles and prayer services. We might not always speak correctly, and even though it appears that our minds are in another place, that doesn't mean that we can't hear the sacred messages or comprehend them at our own level. Give us gentle support when needed, but let us participate and share.

One of the things that I undertook in the last few years before Dad's death was researching our family history and writing his life story. I am starting to do the same for myself. I forget who said it, but "...a spiritual crisis for those with dementia is 'who will carry my story when I am no longer able to do so?'" It's important to us. I hope our grown up kids get involved in this. A fellow parishioner could help someone with dementia write their life story as an individual ministry.[4]

Alzheimer's disease and other forms of dementia wreak havoc throughout our brains, and much of our physical and mental functionality, but not our spirit, not our soul, not the hill within us where the Lord hides, not our special ways of communicating with God/Allah. There's no evidence that our fundamental faith in a supreme being, the one who nurtures us through life and death, has been destroyed or even weakened by this disease. "At least in the early and mid-stages of these diseases, our short term memories are likely impacted; our speech might be impaired. Our spiritual core, often termed one's soul, where we cradle our belief in God/Allah, does not leave the body when we experience Alzheimer's disease. But skills of church ministers for understanding the special faith journey of the person with AD must find new forms of expression in order to be a factor in the lives of those of us who have a cognitive challenge" (Ellor and Sherr 2003).

BE NOT AFRAID

You shall cross the barren desert,
but you shall not die of thirst.
You shall wander far in safety
though you do not know the way.
You shall speak your words in foreign lands
and all will understand.
You shall see the face of God and live.
Be not afraid.
I go before you always.
Come, follow me, and I will give you rest.
If you pass through raging waters in the sea,
you shall not drown.

---

4 *Editors' note:* For a guide on how to write a life story, see Morgan, R. (2002) *Remembering Your Story: Creating Your Own Spiritual Autobiography.* Nashville, TN: Upper Room Books.

If you walk amid the burning flames,
you shall not be harmed.
If you stand before the pow'r of hell
and death is at your side,
know that I am with you through it all.
Be not afraid.
I go before you always.
Come, follow me, and I will give you rest.
Blessed are your poor,
for the kingdom shall be theirs.
Blest are you that weep and mourn,
for one day you shall laugh.
And if wicked tongues insult and hate you
all because of me,
blessed, blessed are you!
Be not afraid.
I go before you always.
Come, follow me, and I will give you rest.

(John 6.20; Isaiah 43.2–3; Luke 6.20; Catholic hymn by Bob Dufford, SJ, based on these scriptures)

Reference

Ellor, J.W. and Sherr, M. (2003) 'God never forgets: Senior ministry and dementia.' Baylor University, Waco, TX.

WORSHIP SERVICES

CHAPTER 1

THE PERSONHOOD OF THE CLERGY

Be Open. Be Humble. Be Adaptable. And Definitely Laugh!

Rev. Theresa M. Brion (Episcopal)

I am a full-time chaplain for a nonprofit religious-affiliated continuing care retirement community (CCRC). My community includes approximately 500 residents, 400 staff, and the family members of both groups of individuals. Thus, I am responsible for attending to the pastoral and other needs of a large community that, although predominantly aged 80 or older, is a rather diverse one in terms of age, education, culture, national origin, and experience. Much of my time is devoted to "serious" matters like running the chapel, leading religious services and spirituality groups, and ministering to the spiritual needs of the community both in life and in death. Fortunately, I have a strong legal, editorial, and business background, which assists me in attending to matters comparable to those of a corporate-sized church. I take seriously the importance of offering a sense of order, calm, and liturgical reverence for the community. Even though it plays to my skills and strengths, delivering this program with compassion and cheer is undoubtedly a challenge. Despite my managerial background and experience, it is my role as chaplain to the residents experiencing increasing or significant dementia, including Alzheimer's disease, that frees my soul and offers me release. In this role I am the wispy and coordinated ballet dancer who also can break out into a Gracie Allen comedic routine with great ease and a hint of a smile. Let me tell you what I mean, for I greatly love what I do as a CCRC chaplain. As I tell others who remark about the joy that radiates from my face, this is the most difficult and yet also the most fulfilling role I have ever assumed in my ministry.

Serving a CCRC community means that I have a deep relationship with the people whom I serve. It frequently is a very intimate relationship, where I know the residents' deepest fears, their greatest joys, and some of the most intimate details of their lives, including their health-care needs, their family dynamics, and the sources of their beings: their remembered selves.

I am thinking of not just what feeds their souls, but how they still envision themselves and attempt to live this out, even if that isn't evident to others. It is a joy and an honor to be invited into that place of intimacy. I am invited to become acquainted with who they are—and it is very important that I use the present tense, for the former colonel or chief executive officer who now depends on others for several activities of daily living or who cannot remember what she ate that morning is still that colonel or chief executive officer. Each person has accomplished so very much, from household to military, from corporation to agency. They have dignity and grace. They are not children, even if their dementia now means that they enjoy "dress up" or coloring and can no longer make their own legal and health-care decisions. The mantra from the movie *The Help*, "You is kind, you is important, you is smart," is a great reminder to me that, yes, they are important and they are smart, but the truly best part is that they also are some of the kindest, most gracious people with whom I have ever worked. They are so appreciative of all things and peoples. They are so accepting of me when I stumble or fail. They also are more than willing to share from their own rich fountain of knowledge if and when it can be helpful.

Be open.

I began this article with the advice "*Be open*" because being open is at the very core of being a chaplain to and with persons experiencing dementia or similar difficulties. Be open to the possibilities of many surprises. On Sundays, another clergy person and I visit with the health-care center residents to bring them communion and check in with them. During that time, we assess changes since we last visited with them, offer them communion, and ask them if they wish to attend our Sunday afternoon mini-service after lunch. We can walk with those who have rollators or walkers (or are just plain confused) and push those who are wheelchair-bound. This requires that both of us and the two or three residents who assist us be open to the possibilities and to change.

Many times, the residents have changed their minds in the 45 minutes since we have asked them and no longer wish to attend the service. Even more of them have forgotten. Some are now taking a nap. Some are still enjoying their dessert or coffee, so we will need to allow them time to finish. Another resident will say no but might be persuaded to come by our suggesting, "Let's give it a try!" Her face will then brighten to a broad grin and she will agree. Some will express a concern that is easily remedied—like borrowing a wheelchair for the weary or assuring that I will get him or her back in time for their expected visitor. If they still decline the offer to attend the service, I gracefully accept their decision without trying to guilt them with my disappointment. Further, I never bring them to the service without their permission.

Be open. Be humble.

My most profound learnings have been from these wise but admittedly confused elders. They look at life so simply and with such great appreciation, making me realize that food, shelter, and family or friends are all that we need. During one Bible study class, I made a colorful Thank You card that I then signed, photocopied, and distributed as part of the lesson of the day. One of the women in our class was so grateful for this simple gesture that she held it close to her chest and thanked me profusely. I felt bad that I had not at least signed each one personally. A simple half-a-cent copy and ten minutes of time yielded such an amazing outcome. Because I know that this particular resident receives regular visits from her attentive family members, it makes me wonder and perhaps worry about the few who receive only infrequent visits because of distance and limited family or friends. The lessons that I learn about gratitude and the importance of sharing one's thankfulness with others for all they are and do is truly invaluable!

Be open. Be humble. Be adaptable.

The Bible studies and health-care center services that I lead require considerable flexibility and adaptability. I am blessed to work with another clergy person who understands that we cannot script these encounters. We never know if we will have five or 15 (or more) for a Bible study or service. We never know if they will be sleeping or responsive, be talkative without regard to the activities in process, or be totally on task.

Some are deaf and cannot follow where we might be in the service or study. Some are unable to respond verbally but will follow along and nod their heads if I sit beside them for singing or whenever else I can and run my finger along the music or other written page. I may need to wake up a resident to offer communion.

Someone may be confused but demand that she be allowed to intinct (dip) the wafer into the small chalice instead of my doing it for her;

however, when I hold the tipped chalice before her, she throws it into the chalice like she had dunked a basketball through the hoop as she gleefully exclaims, "I did it, didn't I?" With a laugh, I join her in her joy and exclaim, "Yes, you did!" Jesus was present with us in our delight, even if a purist might say that she did not receive the Holy Sacrament—a conclusion with which I would disagree. She certainly participated in the sacrament of love and acceptance, didn't she?

We frequently begin our services late or are interrupted by late comers. My Bible study topic may soon morph to another topic based on a resident's response to a particular song or reading. More often than not, the discussion goes a direction that I did not plan. God is present, deciding where we need to be, and that is good. God knows what we need to discuss, and we all know that each of these residents needs to be heard. In the outside world, far too few people take time to sit, listen, and appreciate what our elders might wish to share. What a waste of such rich knowledge and experience!

Adaptability also is key to having a service or study that fits with the attention spans of the residents. We use an abbreviated worship service that includes three or four familiar seasonal hymns on a single song sheet, a brief reading, prayers, and communion. We distribute three pieces of paper: a song sheet; a liturgy sheet; and the brief Bible reading. Each time that we switch between sheets, we go from person to person to make sure that they are at the right place on the correct sheet. Our pianist knows not to begin playing a hymn until everyone is oriented again. The volunteers sit beside one or two residents and assist them as needed. The full service is immediately after Sunday lunch and takes no more than 25 minutes.

My Bible study usually includes a handout or display of colorful pictures or perhaps items that they can see or touch. The study begins with a familiar song and ends with another song, as selected by the residents from a songbook that accompanies a CD with the vocals. The actual lesson takes no more than 20 to 25 minutes. Because the residents have limited short-term memories, they often choose the same songs week after week, and many of our themes revolve around the holidays and popular themes like faith and love. I also must adapt to changing emotions and energy levels, not to mention illnesses and deaths that change the group's dynamics. A disappointing day may mean that the ordinarily perky resident will be quiet or grumpy or even absent. Bible studies and services sometimes compete with family visits and special resident outings.

Be open. Be humble. Be adaptable. And definitely laugh!

Being a chaplain means having a good sense of humor. It also means being sufficiently self-assured to be silly and to laugh at one's self. I am quite petite, so being the silly, perky chaplain is my persona when appropriate. If the boom box is playing show tunes when I come to join the residents for Bible study, I might start dancing and whirling around the room as I enter. If I am leading a line of rollators and wheelchairs as I push a wheelchair back to a room, we might joke about doing a line dance or a train as I skip back to the neighborhoods where they live.

As chaplains and clergy, we frequently hear that we must not share about ourselves since we are to be listeners. However, when leading a Bible study, it is the personal vignette that makes me real and invites others to think of their own stories to share. Some may talk about their military experience or their pets, but they feel open also to sharing their fears as military officers, mothers, wives, friends, when I share from my own experience. I admit my mistakes. I apologize. When one resident with great precision shared that she did not understand what I had said because I failed to speak distinctly, the other staff present behind her quietly laughed as I apologized for my failure. With the critique coming from a former performer and stenographer, she was "right" to note my less than precise diction as one who identifies as Appalachian descent.

So to truly enjoy and reap the rich blessings of this work, a CCRC chaplain must remember to *Be open. Be humble. Be adaptable. And definitely laugh!*

Buddhist Chaplaincy and Dementia

Loving Kindness, Latin Prayers, Chewed Hearing Aids, and the Nature of Impermanence

Chaplain Gillian Renault (Buddhist)

I am a hospice chaplain. My religious life began in a small Protestant church in the south of England. I went to Catholic schools and fell in love with the ritual. As a young adult I embraced Eastern religions, and in the decades since have studied Buddhism (Zen and Vipassana), and Vedanta, as taught by the Hindu monk Swami Vivekananda.

After immigrating to the United States, I turned all my attention to my career, first in journalism, then in the high-pressure world of public relations. Years later, when my mother and then my father died, my career began to feel like a pointless burden. I started working less, volunteered once a week for a nonprofit hospice, and after a few years attended a week-long residential seminar, "Being with Dying," led by Buddhist teacher Roshi Joan Halifax, PhD. My intent was to deepen my volunteer work. Little did I know that those seven days would change my life. The following year I became a student in Dr. Halifax's Upaya Zen Center's Chaplaincy Program.[1] Two years later I graduated and got ordained, ready to start a new career as a hospice chaplain with the Upaya evening chant ringing in my ears.

Let me respectfully remind you,
Life and death are of supreme importance.
Time passes swiftly and opportunity is lost.
Let us awaken. Awaken!
Take heed, do not squander your life.

From Dogen Zenji, 1200–1253 CE

Now I work for the Los Angeles division of a large hospice provider. My mission is to alleviate suffering. I minister to people of all faiths and

1 www.upaya.org

no faith. As the ancient Hindu text, the *Rig Veda*, stated thousands of years ago: "Truth is one; sages call it by various names." Many of our patients have late stage Alzheimer's or other types of dementia. This type of disease doesn't spare patients or families emotionally or spiritually. It is cruel and relentless. It robs patients of their personalities, their speech and understanding, their mobility, and their ability to feed themselves and control their bodily functions. People with end stage dementia can no longer go to church and their families are often too stressed to bring church to them. One of our roles as hospice chaplains is to reconnect them with their spiritual life. Each patient has a unique relationship with God and spirit, as the following case histories demonstrate. The patients' names have been changed, along with minor details of their stories, in order to honor their privacy.

When I met Catherine, she was living in the memory-impaired wing of a Catholic assisted living facility. Sitting in her wheelchair in her room, she was always happy to chat. The rhythm of her speech was still intact, but her conversation consisted of word salad and a few unconnected phrases. Catherine's family told me she was a devout Catholic but she no longer attended mass in the facility's chapel because she didn't understand what was going on. At each visit I would say the *Hail Mary* and play Andrea Bocelli's *Ave Maria* on my iPhone. (iPhones and YouTube are a blessing for chaplains. A quick search and we can access countless prayers, hymns, and music.) Her expression would show a glimmer of recognition, I thought. But that was only my interpretation. How could I tell, really? The rest of the visit I would listen to her, agree with her when the tone of her voice indicated it, talk about the curtains in her room when she gestured toward them, and assure her she was safe when she looked worried or afraid. One afternoon I started to play the *Ave Maria*, as usual, and she suddenly looked at me in delight, her eyes wide. "I haven't heard that in a long time," she said. I was amazed. I had never heard her make such a clear, declarative statement. We listened together and later that day I called her family to tell them what had happened. They too were in awe. Catherine hasn't said anything like this since, having reverted to her word salad conversations. But I still play the *Ave Maria* at every visit.

Buddhism is a vast and diverse philosophy, but consistent to all branches are the Four Noble Truths: Suffering exists. Suffering has an origin and a cause. There is cessation of suffering and there is a Path to alleviate suffering. The way to ease Catherine's suffering—if only for a few moments—emerged that afternoon.

Other Buddhist teachings that influence my work include the loving kindness practice: "May all beings be safe, may all beings be happy, may all beings be free from suffering." Christians see death as a homecoming, and therefore a happy occasion for the deceased, even when those left behind are grieving. For some people, even those with strong faith, death is too frightening to contemplate, but most will agree that feeling safe, and living as happily and free from pain as possible before we die, is a desirable thing, regardless of one's religious beliefs.

Another core teaching of Buddhism is the nature of impermanence. Everything in our current existence is "transient, evanescent, inconstant." Nothing lasts, everything decays and no one can escape sickness, old age and death. Alzheimer's disease is devastating evidence of this doctrine. Its progress may be slow but a patient's condition is likely to change between visits, if only subtly. Families may respond differently at each visit as they come to terms with their loved one's disease and the intense care it requires. Patients and families may question their faith, rely on it more fully, or leave it behind altogether during this time. By embracing impermanence as chaplains, we can be present without expectations, remaining open to whatever is happening that day, in that moment.

The Buddha respected people's desire to practice their own faith, or no faith. This is beautifully expressed in the Dalai Lama's 2012 book, *Beyond Religion: Ethics for a Whole World.* Our role as chaplains is not to convert or persuade people to believe what we believe. Many patients say they are spiritual but not religious. In those cases, we explore what being spiritual means to them: being in nature, perhaps, listening to music, meditating, or being with family and friends. In those cases, worship becomes something apart from church or synagogue—it is whatever lifts up a person spiritually and emotionally. Something that, for at least a few moments, feels more present than their disease.

Angelica is a 90-year-old Filipino woman who knows very little English and is non-verbal most of the time. She lives in a one-bedroom apartment with her daughter-in-law, and her son who has a disability. A hired caregiver attends to her during the day. She has advanced Alzheimer's and spends her days and nights in a hospital bed in the small bedroom, surrounded by large plastic boxes where the family's clothes and other belongings are kept. The television at the foot of her bed plays soap operas and game shows, all in Tagalog.

Our admission records listed her religion as Catholic, but when I visited I saw no icons or pictures of Catholic saints in the apartment. I had to figure out what was important to her spiritually and then offer comfort. Angelica's daughter-in-law worked during the day so I rarely saw her. When I visited I relied upon the Zen Peacemaker tenets of *not knowing* (not assuming the position of expert), *bearing witness* (observing and attuning), and *compassionate action*.[2] I would sit next to Angelica's bed, resting in a place of not knowing. I would speak gently and quietly to her, or as quietly as I could given the frantic dialogue emerging from the TV game shows. I didn't ask to have the television turned off because I didn't want to cause her distress by changing her environment. I felt the answer would emerge. And it did. On my third visit, the hired caregiver told me about Angelica's love of traditional Filipino dance. She used to dance with a group, the caregiver told me, indicating the plastic boxes that contained her costumes.

I pulled up YouTube on my iPhone, did a quick search, and found a video of women performing a Filipino dance. I began to play it, using my small Bluetooth speaker to enrich and amplify the sound. Angelica watched and listened, lying as usual on her back. Suddenly she raised her arms and began to move her hands in a graceful dance. Her fingers were supple and expressive, the movements becoming more elaborate as the minutes passed. The dance ended and I pulled up another video with the same reaction. There was a light in her eyes that hadn't been there before—a sense of connection with the dance. Her arms and hands knew what to do, even if her declining brain couldn't find the words to speak.

Was this worship? One Christian writer defines worship as "a matter of the heart expressed through a lifestyle of holiness." For Angelica, dance that honored her native country's traditions was a matter of the heart. I believe it was holy for her and I could see in her eyes that these videos made her happy. As chaplains we cannot treat or halt the disease process. None of us can. But hopefully we can discover what connects a patient to something beyond her failing body, beyond the bed rails and the humiliating adult diapers, the walls and the ceiling she has looked at for days, weeks, or months. To me, this connection is worship.

2 Founded in 1996, the Zen Peacemakers order is a global organization of socially engaged Buddhists (www.zenpeacemakers.org).

When I met Ernesto and his wife, they were living in a third-floor apartment in a poorly maintained building. Ernesto's diagnosis was end stage Alzheimer's. He and his wife were Catholic. On the walls of the immaculately clean apartment hung pictures of our Lady of Guadalupe and framed prayers in Spanish. The television was tuned to a Spanish talk show. The bedroom was bright and sunny. Ernesto was lying in a hospital bed, gently covered with fresh white sheets with flowers on the hem. He was a handsome man who could still say a few brief sentences in both Spanish and English and would reach out politely to shake a visitor's hand.

Like Angelica, he had already spent weeks in bed. Luckily for him, his wife was an extraordinary woman. After more than 30 years of marriage they still told each other they loved each other, often in my presence. She took wonderful care of Ernesto and was a wealth of information about his life and his many accomplishments. She told me he went to seminary in his native Colombia but never became a priest. "He knows the *Lord's Prayer* in Latin," she told me proudly one day. That was the window I needed to connect Ernesto to his God. I pulled up the audio of the *Lord's Prayer* in Latin, spoken by a man so that Ernesto would be on familiar ground. I also played the *Ave Maria*, sung in Latin by Andrea Bocelli. During the first few visits, Ernesto was able to say the *Lord's Prayer* in Latin along with the recording and to sing the opening lines of the *Ave Maria*, his eyes closed. He always thanked me in English.

As the weeks went by he could remember fewer and fewer words of the Latin *Lord's Prayer*. We tried it in Spanish. He could remember some of it, but each visit I noticed that his brain had robbed him of more words. I stopped playing the prayer in either Latin or Spanish when I realized his wife's encouragement, "Ernesto, say the words, say the prayer," seemed to be causing him distress. However much his wife wished otherwise, the words were no longer available to him. So instead I would ask his wife: "If we were to say a prayer, what would you like to pray for?" "Good health," she would often say. So we would pray for Ernesto's good health. Sometimes denial can ease the pain of inevitable loss.

Every patient and family is unique in the way they connect with their faith and their God, especially when dementia strikes. For the women and men serving as clergy and spiritual caregivers, here are a few things I've learned about caring for these courageous families:

- When visiting a person's home for the first time, do a visual assessment. Are there religious icons or pictures on the wall? If there's a bookcase in view, what titles are there? Even if this person is in your congregation, it's helpful to know how their faith manifests in their home.
- Ask the family and/or the nursing staff at the facility about the patient, his history, his faith, his likes and dislikes. Books she's read. Music she used to enjoy. Even if the person has been a regular member of your congregation, you may discover new information that will help you provide a meaningful worship experience for them. Keep it simple.
- Kerry Egan, a hospice chaplain and author of *On Living* (2016), writes that most of her patients don't talk about God. Instead they talk about their families. Connection with family can be a holy experience, even if it's only through photos. Are there family photos around the house? Show the patient the photos and see if they respond. Ask questions about the people in the picture. Watch for their facial expressions. Don't hurry. Wait, watch, and listen.
- Ask about the patient's favorite hymns or prayers. One dementia patient, a Catholic nun, hadn't spoken but a few words for months—the hospice nurse described her in the chart as non-verbal—but something inspired me to ask her what her favorite hymn was. "Holy God, We Praise Thy Name," she said, clear as a bell. I played it for her, holding the iPhone close to her ear because she was severely deaf. She sang the first verse, every word of it, loudly and profoundly off key. She hadn't spoken this many words in months. She never responded to the question or the hymn again. But that one time she was able to worship her God with gusto.
- Don't assume that a dementia patient's lack of response is always the result of their disease. Many older patients are hard of hearing and, in nursing homes especially, hearing aids can get lost during room changes or mistakenly gathered up with soiled sheets. One facility nurse said our patient had tried to eat her hearing aids, thereby destroying them.

- Music is a profound way to connect with patients spiritually. The nonprofit Music and Memory[3] has demonstrated this many times over. The organization donates iPods, iPhones, or iPads with personalized playlists to dementia patients in nursing homes. The results have been significant and deeply moving. One patient, a retired Christian pastor, hadn't spoken in months and seemed depressed and withdrawn. When he heard the hymns and religious music of his younger days, he became animated and began to interact with other residents. The documentary *Alive Inside* (Rossato-Bennett 2014) chronicles the amazing results for this patient and many others.
- Dementia patients deserve dignity and respect. They are not children, although they often seem like it. A patient's soul and spirit is still whole and perfect. In the early stages of her disease she probably experienced intense frustration, sadness, anger, confusion, and fear. We may not see these emotions in the end stage of her disease, but it's good to remember that she has traveled a long and difficult road. Be kind. Be compassionate. Be sure your body language is open and accepting, the tone of your voice respectful and welcoming. Smile.
- Remember the caregivers. In late stage Alzheimer's it is the family and hired caregivers who experience the frustration and sadness. Mildred was 97 and bed-bound when I started visiting her. She slept most of the day and when awake was non-verbal and combative at times. Her only immediate relatives, a son and his family, lived out of state. Her hired caregiver Doris, however, had lived in Mildred's condo five days a week for eight years. Mildred and Doris were both Christians. Doris asked to have a priest visit and pray for Mildred, even though we both doubted she would understand. It was important to Doris to honor her friend's faith but it was also clear that the priest's prayers, and my visits, were as much for Doris as for Mildred. When Mildred died, Doris grieved deeply.

Hospice provides care through the work of interdisciplinary teams: physician, nurse, home health aide, social worker, chaplain, and perhaps a volunteer coordinate care together. The physicians and nurses work

3 www.musicandmemory.org

diligently to relieve our patients' physical pain, the aides provide personal care, and social workers are a comforting presence for scared and anxious families. Alleviating spiritual suffering and facilitating worship is the work of the chaplain, although it's often the patients and families themselves who show us how. All we have to do is be patient, listen, observe, and respond with compassion.

May I move toward others freely and with openness.
May I receive others with sympathy and understanding.
May I move toward the suffering of others
with peaceful and attentive confidence.
May I recall the Bodhisattva of Compassion, Kwan Yin; her 1,000 hands,
her instant readiness for action, each hand with an eye in it,
the instinctive knowing what to do.
May I continually cultivate the ground of peace for myself and others and
persist, mindful and dedicated to this work, independent of results.

Excerpted from "Meditation on Metta" by Zen teacher Maylie Scott (1994)

References

The Dalai Lama (2012) *Beyond Religion: Ethics for a Whole World.* Tamilnadu, India: Marina Books.

Egan, K. (2016) *On Living.* New York: Riverhead Books.

Rossato-Bennett, M. (dir.) (2014) *Alive Inside.* DVD.

Scott, M. (1994) 'Meditation on Metta.' Retrieved from www.upaya.org/2012/08/metta-prayer-by-maylie-scott on November 02, 2018.

Being with Alzheimer's

Rev. Tim Langdell (Ecumenical Catholic Priest and Zen Buddhist Priest)

Like most ordained Christian pastors, I find my faith gives me vital resources in my work as a hospice and palliative care chaplain. But it is my practice as a Zen Buddhist Priest that makes the job possible for me. Indeed, I would go further and say that Zen practice can be uniquely helpful to anyone working with Alzheimer's patients.

In Zen we have what we call "Beginner's Mind," or "Don't Know Mind." It is this goal of seeking to always be in a state of not-knowing that is such a perfect fit for chaplaincy in general (being a ministry of providing patients with a non-anxious, non-threatening presence) and working with Alzheimer's patients in particular.

Whether we realize it or not—and more often we don't—we enter every situation with a huge number of preconceptions. In general, these help us in everyday life, so there is a good reason we have developed them. If we did not have the concept of a red hot burner on a stove as being dangerous to touch, we might touch it every time and be surprised when it burns us. But these preconceptions are often far more subtle than that, and cause us to miss what is right in front of us, and lead us to be unable to be truly in the moment, fully present to the patient we are visiting.

A quick thought experiment may help us to understand how what we "think" we know about the world stops us in some fundamental ways from actually perceiving the world as it is. Imagine entering a room with brightly colored, floral-patterned wallpaper on every wall. Walk to the center of the room and look straight forward. Now, without moving your eyes or your head from side to side, would you say you are in a room in which you are surrounded by colored wallpaper on all sides? Most people will say yes, and wonder why I asked the rather obvious question! Well, the reality is that you can only see color with the center of your eyes—you cannot see color in the periphery of your vision, let alone outside of your field of vision. We see through rods and cones in our eyes, with the cones being mainly in the very center of the eye and with which we see colors. Rods, on the other hand, are more concentrated toward the edges of our visual field and help us perceive movement.

You can test this for yourself another way: have someone slowly move an object of one distinct bright color from the back of your head to the front. Keeping your eyes focused forward, you will first become aware of the object's presence from the movement but will not at this stage be able to make out its form or its color. Only when it comes right in front of you will you see its color. So, in that room full of brightly colored, floral wallpaper, do we see it as only colored directly in front of us, with the rest of the room monochromatic gray? No, of course not. Our brain fills in the information we cannot see in the moment and constructs a fully colored room around us.

You may feel that this tendency for the brain to "make up" what we are seeing has little to do with our interaction with patients and families. But, have you ever gone into a crowded place and for a moment felt sure you recognized a familiar face? Perhaps you have even started to speak to someone thinking they were someone you know, only to realize it is a stranger? Or perhaps the opposite has happened to you where someone who clearly knows you stops you in the supermarket and starts chatting, but you can't begin to recall who they are. Then, you gradually realize who it is and that you didn't recall them at first because the setting is so different from where you usually see them.

Alzheimer's may be one of the saddest conditions of all, since you lose your loved ones before you lose them to death. In some cases, years before they pass physically, the person you knew and loved has all but disappeared, leaving the visual appearance of someone you knew well and who knew you well, with whom you shared so many memories. This very real grief—for the loss of your loved one as you knew them—can be exceptionally subtle and, understandably, deeply confusing and frustrating.

Early in the progress of the condition there can be merit in helping the person with Alzheimer's to recall what they are forgetting. I have lost count of the number of homes of Alzheimer's patients with notes pinned around the house saying things like "Your name is Mary; this is your house you were born and raised in. Your husband's name is Ron..." and so on. In many instances, after a time this practice becomes more about the family trying to remind the patient for their benefit rather than the patient's benefit. As the patient loses their ability to recollect, it may well be that they are blissfully unaware of the facts, and it is the family who, experiencing this "loss before loss," tries to hold on to any vestige they can of the patient still being who they were. Indeed, it will usually be characterized as the patient not recalling who they are (now) rather than who they were (before).

But often it is not only counterproductive, but perhaps rather unkind to the patient to keep correcting them. To keep "reminding them" of facts that they have no recollection of and do not understand they are getting "wrong." I recall one patient in particular, a 90-year-old lady who enthusiastically greeted me on my chaplain visit as her nephew from Australia (I'm British by birth, by the way, not Australian). She proceeded to tell me that she was born and raised in the Midwest and that her family had come out to California one summer to see the boats and decided to stay. She had an entire life history, which she told me about. And having told me once, she would then introduce herself again as if I had just walked in the room, and tell me the whole history again.

We got on like a house on fire (as they say), discussing the finer points of the boats we have both known and loved (I actually really dislike going on boats as my family will attest!), and our shared memories of growing up in the Midwest (where I have rarely ever been). The patient told me of her deep Catholic faith and asked me to pray with her, which I did. The patient's spirits were substantially lifted.

As I left, her daughter went out of her way to apologize profusely for what her mother had said, adding that her mother was in fact born in the house we were standing in, had never been to the Midwest, and does not have a nephew living in Australia (or anywhere else). She also added that her mother was born and raised Methodist and prior to the onset of Alzheimer's had only bad words to say about the Catholic faith. Puzzled that her mother was now in such good spirits after my visit, she asked what my secret was. And my answer was that I was merely present with her mother, accepting her and what she said in the moment, meeting her right where she is, not where I would prefer her to be or believe she "should" be.

The daughter responded that she had always understood it was wrong to feed her mother's "fantasies" (as the family termed them), and that it was her obligation as her daughter to keep reminding her of the truth of her upbringing, her family, and of her religious faith. Indeed, this is why it is often far easier for a caregiver—be that a chaplain, or nurse, or whomever is involved in the care—to speak with an Alzheimer's patient than it can be for a loved one who is coming from a place of "knowing" that the patient is "wrong" in their memory.

It can be *tremendously* hard for a loved one to put aside the temptation to continually correct an Alzheimer's patient and instead just "be" with the patient, going along with whatever they say. And, certainly, if the condition extends to the patient not recognizing the loved one, or mistaking them for someone else, then it can be exceptionally challenging to just be in the moment and go with whatever is said, whatever happens. Yet if one can successfully make this transition, it can be substantially less stressful and anxiety provoking for both the patient and the family member.

Moreover, on visiting a patient with Alzheimer's, when a family member offers to give me background and tell me about the things the patient will say that are not true, I gently and politely ask that they not do so. As a stranger to the patient, I can be most fully present with them in the moment, and thus be of maximum help, if I am not constantly making assumptions or judgments about what the patient is saying or what I think they will say next.

Before we stray too far from the example I gave above, was it somehow "wrong" of me to join in with a Catholic prayer with a patient who the family says was a dyed-in-the-wool Methodist who disliked Catholicism? I would say a resounding *no*, although I would also understand if some would hold the view that it is theologically or ethically questionable to do so. In that moment this patient sought comfort from a prayer from a faith tradition she was clearly very familiar with, but which she had forgotten she disliked. My role as a chaplain is to meet the patient where they are in that moment, determine their needs in that moment, and do what I am able to meet those needs.

How, then, can we as spiritual counselors or caregivers work on our ability to be a true non-anxious, non-threatening presence for an Alzheimer's patient? How may we get into this "Beginner's Mind" or help family members and others to do so?

On the face of it, it sounds easy, doesn't it, to just "be in the moment." But most of us live our lives constantly thinking about what has happened or what will happen, such that very little of our concentration is on this moment. Trying to stop the constant chatter in our heads so that we can relax and just experience what is happening, and be fully present to the person we are with, is far easier to imagine in theory than to actually do it.

Two generally accepted methods to try to get to this Beginner's Mind state are to take time to do silent meditation and to continue doing whatever you are doing but take time to say quietly to yourself from moment to moment "What's this?" and to answer "Don't know." Silent meditation, often also called "mindfulness" practice or, in Christian terms, "centering prayer," is easy to do, although it may seem alien to you at first. Find time in your day to sit quietly somewhere you will not be disturbed. If you can only find five or ten minutes to try this, then that's fine.

If you are able to sit on the floor on a cushion, cross-legged with your back erect, then that is ideal. The best posture is to sit in what is called either full or half lotus, or Burmese style. But, it is equally fine if you can just find a firm but comfortable chair in which you can sit fairly upright, feet parallel and flat on the floor.

If possible, time yourself. Most "smart" phones these days have a timer on them and there are also Apps such as Insight Timer which will not only time the sitting session for you, but start and end the session with a gentle bell sound. When starting out you may wish to set the timer for just five or ten minutes. While a positive side outcome of this practice can be that you feel more at peace and relaxed, the main goal is to actually become even more fully awake in the moment—even more aware than you usually are. So for this reason I don't recommend closing your eyes while you sit, but rather just look about 45 degrees downwards with your eyelids half open.

At first you may find it helpful to focus on your breath to quiet the usual chatter many of us have going on in our heads all day long. Breathing slowly and deeply, you could try counting your breaths, and I advise counting to ten and then starting from one again. Over time, you will find this simple practice can not only help you feel far more calm, but you may find you are better able to be comfortable just "being" in the moment, not questioning or judging what is happening. And it is this state of mind that can be so very helpful to bring to visits with an Alzheimer's patient.

If you need a little more structure in trying these mindfulness exercises, consider using the STOP technique. You can do this literally any time during the day. The "S" stands for Stop: just stop whatever it is you are doing. You can sit down if that is convenient, or even remain standing. Partially close your eyes, or for this exercise you could entirely shut them. The "T" is for Take a few deep breaths. The "O" stands for Observe what is happening in the moment: What are the sounds around you? What do you smell? How are you feeling in that moment? How does your body feel? Try not to judge what you perceive or feel, but rather just take note of it. And finally the "P" stands for Proceed: having observed for a while—it doesn't matter how long, it can just be a couple of minutes—just proceed and go about the next task at hand.

Following this practice can lead to a radical improvement in working with Alzheimer's patients. One reason for this is that in a sense you are mentally adjusting yourself to better fit with their mental state. We chaplains are taught that where possible it is advisable to get ourselves at the same level as the patient when we visit with them. If they are in a bed or a wheelchair, we are advised to find a chair to be able to sit at their level, rather than towering over them as we speak.

A key symptom of Alzheimer's, although it isn't always framed in this way, is that these patients are in a real sense more in the present moment than we usually are. Like a very young child, they may delight in observing something in the room as if they are seeing it for the first time, over and over again. In a child we often talk of this as being a "child's sense of wonder." Perhaps we should see it the same way with our Alzheimer's patients.

By getting more fully present in the moment, we are adjusting ourselves to be a better fit to the Alzheimer's patient's perception of the world. Rather than seeing their perception as "wrong" and ours as "right," we are meeting them where they are. Then it is far easier to "go with the flow" as a patient greets you yet again as if you have just walked in the room, or asks you again who you are, or comments on something in the room yet again as if they've only just noticed it, or repeats some story or phrase they just said, and so on.

There are numerous benefits of taking this approach. You'll find that you spend less time analyzing them, their speech and behavior, how they have changed or deteriorated, speculating on how things may change for the worse, and instead just be in the present moment, enjoying the time you do have with them. So much time that you could have been present with the patient can be lost while dwelling on such analysis, or on frustration with their condition or their lack of mutual memories.

Rather than feeling we have to keep correcting them, this will enable you to be more at ease just speaking with the Alzheimer's patient. If they are not communicating with you, then being present in the moment gives you at least two options: you can be comfortable in your own skin just sitting with them without feeling the need to have to talk; or, if you do talk, tell them about your day or talk about almost anything. You can feel more at ease just to do so without being bogged down in analytical thinking of whether they understand what you're saying, whether what you are doing is benefiting them, or so on. Be assured, just being there, being fully present with them, not correcting them when they say things that are not "true," is most likely benefiting them immensely.

Some may feel uncomfortable when this being in the moment with the patient leads to joining in, or just going along with, the fantasy they are spinning. To some this may seem wrong, as if it is feeding a problem that should not be encouraged. On the contrary, communicating with someone with Alzheimer's is an invitation to enter into their reality. Practicing this Don't Know Mind, putting aside what you think you know about the patient, can help immensely with more fully entering into their reality—as at odds as it may be with yours.

Thus if the patient is convinced their spouse is still alive, or if they talk as if they are a young child and speak of their mother or even their grandmother as still alive (all of which I have witnessed on several occasions), then if it is not harming anyone, to the extent possible enter into this reality with them. Avoid the temptation to correct them. Coming from a Beginner's Mind perspective, this is far easier than coming from a knowing mind full of what "ought" to be the case. This approach should also make it easier for you to resist the temptation to finish the Alzheimer's patient's sentences for them and instill in you a greater patience and sense of being in their time, not the world's time you usually participate in.

If you have worked with Alzheimer's patients before, then you will know to keep distractions in the environment to a minimum. But what being more centered in the moment can also help you with is sensing more swiftly when the patient's mood may change, which is not unusual with these patients. Sensing they may be about to swing from being happy to sad, or from relaxed to anxious or angry, you can more effectively distract the patient, gently, so that the negative emotion or outburst is avoided, or at least lasts less long.

Your key goal here is the comfort and well-being of the Alzheimer's patient, to provide loving, compassionate care. You will also find it comes more naturally to make gentle eye contact with the patient, and to keep your tone more moderate and reassuring, never challenging or admonishing.

Again, where possible, encourage two-way communication, but if they do not wish to speak or cannot speak, do feel free to continue to speak to them and never talk as if they are not present. Some sources advise you to just keep talking no matter what, but an advantage of coming from this Don't Know Mind space of being centered in the moment is that you are better able to determine if the moment is right to keep talking, or if the patient will prefer just to sit in silence for some moments, maintaining eye contact, and perhaps holding hands.

Lastly, use these centering and mindfulness techniques to help with self-care. Working with an Alzheimer's patient can be stressful. The same meditation and mindfulness techniques that I have recommended above to help you get into Beginner's Mind—just be in the moment—can also assist in dealing with the stresses and anxieties that arise from working with this patient population.

This article has been written to convey the advantages I have found for using Zen Buddhist practices in working with Alzheimer's patients, and to encourage you to try similar approaches yourself. But, needless to say, do seek out other chaplains or caregivers with similar Zen or mindfulness training to assist in the patient's care where you believe having someone able to be fully present in the moment may help. You'll find that more often than not, it is of great help.

Chapter 2

CONDUCTING SERVICES IN CARE COMMUNITIES

Nurturing the Spirit through Worship

Rev. Kathy Fogg Berry (Interdenominational Christian)

Jim never sits still. Ten years into his dementia journey, he rarely stops walking except to eat meals and sleep. He seems to be on a mission, but only he knows what it is. When devotions begin each Monday afternoon in his memory support household, Jim quite often walks through the group as people are greeted, scriptures are read, and the Lord's Prayer is said. But when everyone joins their voices in singing the old traditional hymns, Jim takes a seat and joins in the choruses. He seems transformed to another time and place that makes sense.

Dorothy faithfully comes to worship each week, but rarely speaks. Due to her advanced dementia, the words no longer flow. But, she loves helping pass out the bulletins and nodding a greeting to people as they arrive. One week, after we all said the Lord's Prayer, Dorothy walked over to me in the middle of worship, grabbed my arm, and began trying to tell me something. "Prayer...prayer...here..." she said after much effort. Pausing a few seconds, she added "all...here," as her arm swept toward the people encircling us. Her eyes bore into mine pleadingly, willing me to understand what she was saying. "Are you talking about the Lord's Prayer, Dot?" I asked. Nodding her head, she continued, "Prayer...all...here." Taking her hand in mine I asked, "Dot, are you saying you enjoy saying this prayer together with everyone here?" As she nodded her head vigorously, her beaming smile said it all.

Worship, corporate or individual, reminds us who we are and whose we are. It anchors us to the source and strength of our lives and gives life meaning. For Jim and Dorothy, and countless people experiencing dementia who've spent much of their lives practicing their faith through worship, continuing to worship remains a vital part of nurturing their spirit.

Dementia causes loss, so much loss. But the spirit lives on, never lost. Words may fail, but the reality of God within us, around us, and sustaining us doesn't. When those living with dementia can no longer worship in ways that might bring them hope, comfort, and peace, when they can no longer initiate faith practices, like worship, which strengthens relationship with God and others, they suffer yet another huge loss. By offering person-centered spiritual care, we can help.

For the past eight years I've been privileged to serve as the memory support chaplain at Westminster Canterbury Richmond, a 900-resident continuing care retirement community in Richmond, Virginia. Westminster Canterbury Richmond was founded by the Episcopal and Presbyterian denominations in 1975, and while it now serves residents of 26 different faith traditions, the majority of residents are Christian. Approximately 130 residents with dementia diagnoses live in three designated memory support areas where weekly worship services and devotions are designed intentionally for people in the early to late stages of dementia. Spiritual support is also offered to families and staff. Residents who have difficulty worshiping in a group are offered one-on-one worship experiences particular to their needs.

Most people living with dementia still thrive on socialization and being in relationship with others. Facilitating worship in memory support areas requires going with the flow, embracing and affirming words and actions which are, at times, impulsive. Inclusion and acceptance are keys to fostering successful worship experiences.

Many chaplains and ministers serve multi-cultural, multifaith memory support communities full of wonderfully diverse worshipers. It may be hard to find common ground even when your population is more religiously homogenous because, as we know, everyone practices faith in unique ways. Tim Ford, a chaplain researcher at Virginia Commonwealth University Medical Center in Richmond, Virginia, is Buddhist, representing the noble Karma Kagyu lineage, a Tibetan denomination. "Buddhism," he says, "is extraordinarily diverse. It is not uncommon for practitioners from different towns, much less different countries, to not recognize others' rituals and devotions. Buddhism is also not very reliant on scripture, especially for lay practitioners; so coming up with universal practices is very challenging" (personal communication).

He suggests, however, that there are common tenets, values, and attitudes that may be of use:

- Equanimity is a universal value as both a mindful presence and a manifestation of love/compassion. Maintaining an attentive and peaceful aspect towards another is considered a deep form of generosity (the first and most fundamental of the primary Buddhist virtues).

- Offering incense is also relatively universal, both as reverence for the space/time/person but also in memory of ancestors, teachers, and/or Archetypal beings. Therefore, scents used as sacred would be very effective clinically. Again, the specific scents vary somewhat, but, for example, "joss sticks" of sandalwood are common to several traditions and heavily used in the West.

- Ringing a clear bell or chime is a popular way to mark sacred time/space. Letting a particularly resonant bell "ring out" into quiet is an excellent sensory invitation to still the mind.

- Bowing is a deep practice unto itself, but again the specific postures vary slightly by region.

- There is also mantra practice, or chanting, which is not universal, but popular in many denominations. The Sanskrit prayer from the Heart Sutra—"Om gate gate paragate parasamgate bodhi svaha"—is probably the most well known of the Buddhist mantras. It roughly translates to: "Gone, gone, gone beyond, gone even beyond that, the enlightened heart and mind are one."

Dr. Sultan Lakhani, a geriatric psychiatrist for Bon Secours Hospitals in Richmond, Virginia, is a life-long Shia Muslim. "Muslims," he says, "learn prayers when they are very young, and they are not forgotten, by most people, even in the end stages of dementia." The prayers, which come from the Quran, "keep them calmer," he says. "The most frequently said prayer is Surah Al Fatiha and contains seven lines recited each day." There are many, slightly different versions of this prayer as each sect may translate or pronounce these words a little differently.

Bismillaah ar-Rahman ar-Raheem
Al hamdu lillaahi rabbil 'alameen
Ar-Rahman ar-Raheem Maaliki yaumid Deen
Iyyaaka na'abudu wa iyyaaka nasta'een
Ihdinas siraatal mustaqeem
Siraatal ladheena an 'amta' alaihim

Ghairil maghduubi' alaihim waladaaleen
Aameen

In the name of God, the infinitely Compassionate and Merciful.
Praise be to God, Lord of all the worlds.
The Compassionate, the Merciful. Ruler on the Day of Reckoning.
You alone do we worship, and You alone do we ask for help.
Guide us on the straight path,
the path of those who have received your grace;
not the path of those who have brought down wrath, nor of those who wander astray.
Amen.

Translated by Kabir Helminsk[1]

Other important spiritual disciplines within the Islamic faith which a person is to do, if he is physically and mentally able, include:

- fasting during the month of Ramadan
- praying three to five times a day, depending on your sect
- eating food that is halal – consistent with Islamic guidelines
- performing the Hajj or pilgrimage to Mecca once in a lifetime
- maintaining a high standard of personal hygiene
- sprinkling holy water on the face as an important act to bring forgiveness of sins.

If a Muslim is not able to do these disciplines, others are to help, Dr. Lakhani says. Prayers can be shortened for the sick, the weak, and the needy. "Hearing the Quran read and prayers recited," he adds, "may spur the memory of someone with a dementia disease and enable him to practice his faith" (personal communication).

Like Buddhism and Islam, Christianity, Judaism, and other religions contain many denominations or sects encompassing differences and similarities in how they express their faith. Common Hindu spiritual disciplines include worship, meditation, pilgrimages, and festivals, but Hindus practice those tenets in thousands of different ways. Each Native American within each Native American tribe practices spirituality

1 https://sufism.org/origins/quran-islam/quranic-chapters/the-fatiha-2

uniquely. And while some Protestant denominations use prayer books in worship, others offer free-flowing prayers. Some Catholics are strictly liturgical, while others are evangelical when expressing their faith.

All of this is to say that planning worship for groups of people in different stages of dementia can be complicated, but worth the effort for the people we serve. Learning each individual's spiritual needs and disciplines leads to discovering the group's common worship ground. Enlisting a priest, rabbi, Imam, or other spiritual leader to assist with corporate or individual worship may be needed. Gathering a group of people, from similar or diverse faith traditions, and focusing on a universal theme can lead to a wonderful sense of community and celebration of life.

Creating a worship environment

Before gathering people for an optimal 20–30-minute worship time, create a welcoming atmosphere. Because most of the residents I serve at Westminster Canterbury are Protestant, I'll highlight preparing for a Protestant service. Other faith traditions can include worship elements, symbols, scriptures, and prayers distinctive to those traditions.

A table is set with linens, candles (battery-operated because of safety regulations), flowers, an open Bible, and a cross. Some services include potpourri to mimic the burning of incense. As residents arrive, independently or in wheelchairs, they hear music, from a volunteer musician when possible. The music is typical of what they would hear upon entering a sanctuary. Even if worship is usually offered in a dining or multi-purpose room, the presence of symbols of faith transforms the makeshift worship space. Upon seeing and hearing these visual and auditory calls to worship, many residents are visibly moved into a spirit of reverence. Often, those who were restless settle down. Furrowed, anxious brows often relax and questioning voices often quiet. As other residents join the semi-circle, there is a sense of peace. People are listening. Invite caregivers and visiting family members to join in, adding to the community of faith.

There will be disruptions and some residents will have difficulty settling down, but quiet greetings and reassurances can help; restless needs can be met and souls touched. As residents gather, I greet them individually by name with a friendly handshake or caress of the arm, reminiscent of how they would have been greeted upon arriving at church. Introducing myself, I welcome each person to our worship time, and introduce them to the person sitting on their right and left, encouraging community. Then I make the service as interactive as possible to actively engage each participant.

Suggested order of service

Invite everyone to say the Lord's Prayer in unison

This prayer, which Christ taught his disciples, is iconic. Interdenominationally, it is recognized and remembered by Christian worshipers. Many people living in the late stages of dementia can recite it even when they can no longer converse. It is powerful and miraculous to hear people, who are often marginalized for what they can no longer do, join together lifting their voices in reverence to God. Saying this prayer together at the beginning of the service establishes a reverent tone and sense of togetherness.

Lead them in reciting a familiar scripture passage

Use scriptures such as Psalms 23, Psalms 118.24, Psalms 100, or John 3.16.

Starting worship with elements which residents can fully participate in establishes community and joy in participation. It connects them not only to the God they're worshiping but to each other in fellowship and unity. They become one worshiping body.

Sing two or three familiar hymns

Select hymns which go with the theme you've selected for the service. Music is a powerful expression of praise and worship, and residents can sing, too, far beyond the time they can converse. Even when they can no longer sing, you'll see toes tapping, hands clapping, and other signs of engagement.

Interactive reflection and scripture

Select a worship theme and scripture to support it. Build the reflection around themes like: love, God's presence, hope, peace, the gift of family, God's creation, etc. Rather than lecturing or sermonizing, share a short (five to ten minute) dialogical reflection asking for comments and reflections from participants. If possible, enlist a resident to read the scripture for the day. When she is finished, affirm her for reading and read the passage again for those who may not have heard.

Sing two or three more hymns

Over the years, our group has chosen to consistently sing one hymn as our final hymn. "In the Garden" elicits such expressions of contentment and peace on their faces. Find what works for your group.

Prayer

Ask for prayer requests before praying. Residents in the early stages of dementia often contribute requests. Listen for responses from people in the middle to late stages, but if they don't come, suggest a few ideas like family, health, friends, or the world. Watch for nods, smiles, or other visual consents. Ask a resident to pray, if you know that is something she's comfortable doing.

Individual blessings

As music plays in the background, visit each resident in the semi-circle, shaking hands or offering a gentle touch. Express thanks for his presence at the service and a blessing. On many occasions I've experienced residents, who'd appeared to be sleeping the entire service, open their eyes when I touched them and respond with things like "This was wonderful," "Bless you, too," and "Thanks be to God." This reminds me that I can never underestimate people's faith experiences or the moving of God's spirit among us.

Continue music as residents disperse

They enjoy listening to or singing along with music as others are assisted back to their households. Often residents continue singing as they're wheeled down the halls and aides tell of them humming or singing the rest of the day.

Theme suggestions

Thanking God for our senses

Within the structure suggested above, provide a devotional thought that appeals to the senses and is interactive, based on John 10.10 where Christ said: "I came that they may have life, and have it abundantly." Explain how God helps us live life abundantly by using the wonderful senses God gave us.

Bring props which represent the five senses for this experiential dialogue. One by one, introduce the items and go around to each individual, letting them smell, taste, see, hear and feel.

- *Smell*—cinnamon, cloves, lavender, orange, coconut, garlic
- *Taste*—cotton candy, citrus, licorice, peppermint, chocolate *(Check for allergies and swallowing issues before serving food)*
- *See*—laminated pictures from calendars, a DVD or video portraying scenery, picture book, different objects
- *Hear*—different styles of music, a noisemaker with sounds of nature, bird calls, music instruments
- *Feel*—conch shell, stuffed animal, soft blanket, sand, pebbles, pine cone.

As you're going around the circle, ask them about each item. Invite people to share with the group what they smell, taste, see, hear, and feel. Affirm and accept each comment.

Join in the following responsive prayer, encouraging residents, visitors, and caregivers to join you in saying "Thanks Be to God" after each statement.

God, we thank you for the gift of sight.
Thanks be to God.
God, we thank you for the gift of touch.
Thanks be to God.
God, we thank you for the gift of hearing.
Thanks be to God.
God, we thank you for the gift of taste.
Thanks be to God.
God, we thank you for the gift of smell.
Thanks be to God.

Thank you, God, for giving us senses and helping us live abundantly.
Thanks be to God!

Suggested hymns

Count Your Blessings

Praise God From Whom All Blessings Flow

Showers of Blessings

Now Thank We All Our God

Joyful, Joyful We Adore Thee

Seeing God in nature

In the spring or summer, have a worship time outdoors, maybe even while taking a walk. Follow the format, selecting hymns on nature and scripture about nature, like Psalm 95. Ask residents to look around and talk about where they see God in nature. How do different objects remind them of God? Have some examples from your own life ready to share. If you can't go outside, bring bits of nature inside: leaves, flowers, rocks, twigs, pine cones, birds' nests. Place them in a bag and let residents take turns pulling one out.

Thankfulness: My favorite things

Within the framework of the suggested order of worship, lead residents in a service of thankfulness at Christmas time, or any time of year. Along with various carols, sing composers Rodgers and Hammerstein's famous song from *The Sound of Music*: "My Favorite Things."

During the interactive reflection time, reveal a medium-sized, wrapped present—top and bottom wrapped individually. Inside the box have strips of paper with one of the following questions written on it: Favorite Christmas carol? Favorite Christmas animal? Favorite Christmas ornament? Favorite Christmas story? Favorite Christmas tree topper? Favorite Christmas activity at Church? Favorite Christmas decoration? Favorite Christmas smell? Favorite Christmas candy? Favorite person to see at Christmas? Favorite Christmas nativity character? Favorite Christmas gift?

Go to each resident and encourage him to select a strip, helping as needed. Let him read it and answer, if possible, then encourage the group to respond to the question. Talk about each strip and engage participants as much as possible. Be prepared to share personal stories from your life that go with each strip. That will prompt memories and reflections from the group. Orchestrate strip selections so that "Favorite Christmas gift?" is selected last. Let this lead to reflecting on thankfulness for all the things mentioned and the greatest gift, Jesus Christ.

Sing "Away in a Manger," "O Holy Night," "Silent Night," and other beloved carols.

Psalms and song

Offer a worship service where you alternate reading from the Psalms and singing old, traditional hymns that go with each Psalm's theme. Invite residents to say the Psalms with you, as they are able.

One-on-one worship experiences

Charles and Ann served communion together for years as Eucharistic volunteers at Westminster Canterbury. Because he's now wheelchair-bound and in the late stages of dementia, Charles can no longer serve with Ann in this meaningful ministry, which is a great loss for both of them. In a group setting, Charles usually sleeps deeply, often snoring loudly. But, in one-on-one worship, Charles responds to the closeness of my voice, gentle touch, and seeing Holy Communion elements. Upon receiving the sacraments he quietly says, "Thanks be to God."

Mary has great difficulty settling down in a group setting. She constantly shifts in her wheelchair and calls out for help during worship. She can't hear what the worship leader is saying and constantly yells, "What are you saying?" Other participants get unsettled by her restlessness and anxiety. When we worship one-on-one, she enjoys holding hands, singing along with encouragement, helping read the scripture, and touching each element of worship. At the end of our times she always says, "Thank you, this has been special."

Agnes was almost always in pain. Arthritis had crippled her hands and feet. Her chin was permanently tucked and her tiny frame was dwarfed by her wheelchair. On top of physical problems, she was in the middle stages of dementia. Not understanding that she could no longer walk, she constantly tried to get out of her wheelchair. To keep her safe, she was often sitting by the noisy nurses' station. Usually she told me to go away, like she did everyone, but one beautiful spring day when I asked if she wanted to go outside, she said, "Yes." Wheeling her outside, I suggested we sit quietly and not talk, allowing the beauty of nature to speak. For 30 minutes we sat and listened to the birds and felt the wind caress our cheeks. At the end of our outside time I simply said, "Thanks be to God," and she said, "Amen."

Knowing each individual's physical, emotional, and spiritual needs can help you create a meaningful experience for one-on-one worship. Invite a family member or friend to join in, if it's appropriate.

Most of the group worship suggestions contained in this article can be adapted for use in one-on-one visits. Facilitating worship is holy, whether corporate or individual. As John Swinton reminds us in his book *Dementia: Living in the Memories of God*:

> If people act toward us in ways that remind us that we are remembered, then we can see, feel, and touch God's memories in action. As we encounter others, we encounter God. If each encounter between human beings is an encounter with the holy, then one vital dimension of God's active memory relates to the ways in which God's people encounter one another. (2012, p.222)

Reference

Swinton, J. (2012) *Dementia: Living in the Memories of God.* Cambridge, UK: William B. Eerdmans Publishing Company.

Worship *With* Rather Than *For*

(Ret.) Bishop Kenneth L. Carder (United Methodist) and Norma Smith Sessions (American Baptist)

> Now there are varieties of gifts, but the same Spirit; and there are varieties of services but the same Lord; and there are varieties of activities, but it is the same God who activates all of them in everyone. (1 Corinthians 12.4–6, *New Revised Standard Version*)

What follows in this article are insights we have gained from our experiences as caregivers of our spouses, Dale and Linda. Dale is a retired American Baptist pastor and a mental health counselor in addiction treatment and long-term care facilities. He is in mid-stage Alzheimer's disease, a disease from which his father and brother died. Linda has a background in Christian education and extensive volunteer involvement with children and older adults. She was diagnosed in 2009 with frontotemporal dementia and is now under hospice care in the severe stage of her disease.

We also bring to the subject professional and academic engagement as a pastor, bishop, and seminary professor and as a MSW social worker with study and experience in gerontology. We regularly co-teach with a hospice chaplain a seminary course entitled "Dementia through a Pastoral Theological Lens." Additionally, we volunteer as chaplain and worship leaders at Bethany, the memory care facility located in the retirement community in which we live. In our volunteer capacity, we lead devotions each Thursday and community worship each Sunday at Bethany.

Worship in a memory care facility takes many forms. A fairly typical service involves a pastor from a local congregation entering the facility, perhaps with a small group of musicians, and proceeding to sing, read Scripture, pray, and deliver a brief homily. Interaction with residents is minimal, and participation by the residents is limited primarily to observation. The worship is done *for* the residents and becomes another activity to entertain the residents.

Liturgy, however, is "the work of the people" and includes the congregation members offering their gifts in adoration, thanksgiving, and dedication to God. Authentic worship is always done *with* members of the congregation, else it is an activity done *to* and *for* the entertainment of the congregation.

Much congregational worship is print-oriented and involves abstract thinking and attentiveness, requiring high levels of cognitive engagement. People in varying stages of cognitive decline tend to live in the moment and language comprehension and expression is limited. These factors combine to marginalize them in a typical worship service.

When a different approach is used, however, people with neuro-cognitive impairments are not only included, but their gifts are incorporated into the worship experience. This approach involves special sensitivity, inordinate flexibility, and spontaneous creativity among worship leaders. An interactive liturgy that focuses on consistency of relationships and the stories and gifts of the worshiping community has the potential to be worship *with*.

Gifts participants bring to worship

People with cognitive impairments bring multiple gifts that contribute to corporate worship. Those gifts emerge as the community gathers for worship. Many need assistance from staff and one another to attend the service. The "gathering" itself is a significant part of the worship as people come arm-in-arm to find their seats. Those with visual and mobility losses are assisted by fellow worshipers and the bond between them is evident.

Preparing the space for worship becomes a communal experience, as staff, residents, volunteers, and family members cooperate in moving chairs. Arranging the altar becomes another shared event as the congregation members arrive for the service. Two women who served as members of their local church "altar guilds" make sure the frontal is straight and the flowers and cross are appropriately placed.

The flowers themselves promote engagement in the experience. The only time live or cut flowers are allowed in the unit is during worship. The responses upon seeing the beauty of nature become sighs of praise: "Those are so pretty." "Beautiful." "May I touch them?" "Are those for me?" "Let me smell them."

Gift of music

One of the most obvious and expressive gifts persons with cognitive impairments bring to worship is music. Music seems to be almost a universal language among those with cognitive impairment. Neuroscientists document that the portion of the brain which retains familiar music diminishes more slowly and is one of the last abilities to be lost.

It is not uncommon for people with very limited recall and little spoken language to sing the lyrics of many hymns. Accessing their reservoir of sung theology creates a work of communal praise and kindles memories that transcend their cognitive limitations.

Music plays a key role in worship at Bethany. Identifying the hymns with which the people there are familiar was the first challenge. The people at Bethany come from a variety of religious backgrounds: Catholic, Lutheran, Baptist, Pentecostal, Episcopal, Presbyterian, United Methodist, and Jewish. Therefore, identifying familiar hymns across the spectrum involved experimentation over time. Of course, some hymns were immediately recognizable: "Amazing Grace," "Jesus Loves Me," "What a Friend We Have in Jesus," "How Great Thou Art," "This Is My Father's World," "In the Garden," "My Faith Looks up to Thee," "Holy, Holy, Holy," "Standing on the Promises," "God Will Take Care of You," and "Blest Be the Tie That Binds." Hymns with refrains are especially appreciated since they provide repetitive words and sounds.

The people at Bethany bring varied levels of musical skills to the worship service. One is a retired music teacher with a beautiful voice. She and her husband, also a resident, sing with gusto, which encourages others to join. Doug is a life-long Lutheran who has been blind since childhood. He knows the lyrics of many hymns and can be counted on to fill in words that others may have forgotten. Each time we sing "Jesus Loves Me," Doug renders a solo on a seldom-sung verse:

Jesus loves me! He who died
Heaven's gate to open wide
He will wash away my sin
Let His little child come in.

Given the stage of life of this congregation, Doug's verse has become especially comforting. They join the refrain with reverence and devotion.

Yes, Jesus loves me
Yes, Jesus loves me
Yes, Jesus loves me
The Bible tells me so.

Conventional understanding assumes that people with dementia can learn nothing new. That doesn't seem to be true when it comes to music, at least in many cases. For example, Deborah, the housekeeper at Bethany, loves to sing as she works. One of her favorites is "This Is the Day." Few, if any, knew the song. We asked Deborah to help lead us in singing it. Now each Sunday's service begins with the chorus as our Call to Worship.

Another hymn Deborah taught and sometimes leads is "Love Lifted Me." It has become a favorite because of the chorus:

Love lifted me!
Love lifted me!
When nothing else could help,
love lifted me.
Love lifted me.

Indeed, the message and mood of the chorus speaks to the deep experiences and longing for loving relationships.

Gift of movement

Music generates a variety of expressions in worship. People with cognitive impairments tend to live in the heart more than the brain, in feelings more than abstract thoughts. Therefore, music in worship generates and expresses feelings more than theological reflection. For some, the feelings are expressed in movements and gestures rather than in singing; and those movements contribute to the corporate experience.

Ethel, for example, loves "Swing Low, Sweet Chariot," even though she never sings the words. Instead, she does liturgical movements with her hands. Her movements are always in time with and related to what is being sung. Her responses to other hymns are similar; she bodily enacts the rhythm and lyrics, thereby contributing immensely to our worship with her gift of movement.

Others respond with more subdued bodily movements—smiles, tapping the feet, gently touching their leg in tempo with the beat, or perhaps a glimmer of joy in the eyes. Yes, and some sleep! But members of the congregation are contributing their gifts in response to God's gift of music.

Gifts of embedded faith practices

The congregation members at Bethany also contribute their gifts of embedded faith practices. The variety of liturgical practices adds to the richness of the worship. Some come from more "free church" traditions where spontaneous verbal responses flow freely. Others have been shaped by formal liturgy and are accustomed to prefacing prayer with "The Lord be with you" and the response "And also with you."

The current generation of older people values reverence in worship. Except those whose disease has destroyed their sense of boundaries, the people at Bethany stop whatever they are doing when the worship service begins. They suddenly offer the gift of silence, when only a few moments before chatter and movement were dominant.

Memory is more than brain. Muscles have memory. Cells have memory. The body is our memory, our past. Images and sounds trigger cognitively forgotten actions. The body seems to remember worship postures and movements. Bowing the head or folding the hands for prayer, for example, seems to be an automatic response to "Let us pray." Inspiration emerges in a community of bowed heads and folded hands in prayer, even if the words of the prayer are incomprehensible. The body prays when the voice and brain cannot.

The Eucharist is an embedded practice that transcends cognitive comprehension, and people with dementia diseases bring a lifetime of participation in this outward and visible sign of an inward and spiritual grace. Lutherans and Episcopalians routinely reach forth their folded and cupped hands to receive the bread. The wondrous look in the eyes and hushed reverence proclaims the mystery of the Sacrament.

Dale regularly assists with serving Communion by sharing the Cup with participants. A person with Alzheimer's serving the Sacrament with people who share the disease is a moving experience for us all. His embedded pastoral practices come to the forefront as he greets worshipers with "God is with you," or "God bless you." He often sits following the service with congregation members, holding their hands to comfort and encourage. Family members and other visitors marvel at Dale's "pastoral presence" even though his verbal and cognitive skills are very limited.

Every person present contributes to the worship experience in some way. Some actively share in each component of the liturgy, dependent upon the stage and/or manifestation of the disease. Others contribute by their mere presence and subtle actions, such as facial expressions, holding the hand of the person seated beside them, nodding the head in affirmation, bowing the head prayerfully.

Worship leadership among people with dementia

Incorporating the spontaneous actions of the members of the worshiping community requires flexibility on the part of the leader. Since the disease has removed boundaries and limited the attention to the present moment, disruptions are commonplace. Someone may suddenly leave her chair and wander about the room or make an incoherent sound. Maintaining focus requires discipline and flexibility on the part of the leader.

Barbara typically walks around during the worship service, which can be a distraction for some. She most frequently stays to herself and is non-verbal and, therefore, doesn't sing the hymns or recite any of the liturgy. Frequently, however, she moves close to the center of the activity. She enjoys standing near the pianist while she is playing and beside the leader as he/she speaks. When she comes beside us as we lead, we put our arms around her and she smiles with genuine appreciation and affection. Worshipers sense the expressed compassion and the sense of community increases.

Worship *with* rather than *for* people who live with dementia diseases requires an interactive liturgy that allows for improvisation. Since the worshipers live in the present moment, the leader must be comfortable in responding to unexpected outbursts or interruptions. Those unplanned interruptions often turn out to be profound experiences of worship.

Pentecost Sunday represented such an unexpected experience. The Scripture Lesson for the day was the story of Pentecost in Acts 2. During the reading of "and there came like the rush of a violent wind," Bobby, who is seldom still or visibly attentive in the service, spontaneously yelled "O, my God!" We paused and replied, "You know, Bobby, I bet there were many at that event who said the same thing. Thank you!"

After describing the diversity of languages, nationalities, and cultures present at the celebration, I said that they still understood one another. "What made that possible?" I asked. Following a few moments of silence, Mary said, "They loved one another!"

There followed a brief statement that God's Spirit is the spirit of love. Knowing that different languages were present among the Bethany congregation, I said, "Love is spoken in different languages. Let's see if we can hear it in other tongues. José, how do you say love in Spanish?"

"Amor," responded José! We then had each participant turn to the person beside them and say, "Amor."

We did the same with each language represented among the staff, residents, family members, and visitors present: Italian, French, German, and Swahili. Barbara, whose language consists of incoherent babbles, stood beside me. I said to the congregation, "Some of us lose language and can't say 'love' in any language. How do we communicate love to Barbara?"

"Hug! Hug her!" was the immediate response from a resident. I put my arm around Barbara, looked into her eyes, and said, "Barbara, I love you!" With a smile that communicated deep understanding and emotion, she replied hesitantly but clearly, "I...love...you!" Pentecost happened at Bethany! The service appropriately concluded with "Blest Be the Tie That Binds."

The rhythm of the liturgical year is embedded in many of the people at Bethany and they respond intuitively to the seasons—Advent, Christmas, Epiphany, Lent, Easter, Pentecost. Colors and music and acts appropriate to the season kindle memories and deeply rooted actions. Special liturgical occasions can become profoundly meaningful, as the experience on Pentecost Sunday demonstrates.

"Baptism of Our Lord Sunday" provides occasion to reawaken the significance of baptism in the lives of people with dementia diseases. An added feature of the worship center on this Sunday was a basin and pitcher, creating curiosity as worshipers gathered. "What is that?" asked one worshiper. "We are going to talk about baptism, and this is water to remind us," I replied.

After reading the story of Jesus's baptism, I talked briefly about the voice from the heavens: "You are my Son, the beloved, and with you I am well pleased." There followed a few minutes of conversation about how God seeks to speak to us the same words: "You are my beloved, son or daughter, and I delight in you."

Some participants shared stories of their own baptism or what they had been told about their baptism by their parents. As expected, some had been immersed as adults; others had been baptized as infants.

Some made no response as though they had no comprehension of what was happening.

After calling attention to the altar, I poured water from the pitcher into the basin, making sure that the sound of water could be heard. With my friend and pastoral colleague Dale holding the basin, we approached each participant. Looking into each person's eyes, I dipped my hand into the water and formed the sign of the cross on the forehead as I called each name: "(Name), you are God's beloved son/daughter. With you God is delighted." The responses ranged from a polite smile and "thank you" to tears of joy and "yes"!

Others watched with eagerness and anticipation as Dale and I went to each participant. Music played in the background. The sounds, the feel of the water on the foreheads, and the verbal and non-verbal responses all became a corporate act of praise and devotion to which each contributed their varied gifts.

Sensory gifts

The worship on Baptism of Our Lord Sunday illustrates the importance of tactile expressions as means of interactive worship. The participants bring to worship a heightened response to sensory stimuli. The sight and smell of fresh flowers elicit positive responses, as do the colors of the paraments.

Appropriate gentle touch sparks memories and manifestations of deeply embedded compassion. Worshipers frequently hold the hand of the person beside them and they react appreciatively to the pastor's clasp of the hand or kind placement of the hand on the shoulder. Following the benediction each week, Dale and I greet each congregant with handshakes and hugs.

The worshiping community at Bethany becomes especially engaged when visuals and objects that can be touched are included. Since our community is made up of persons whose capacity for abstract thinking has been diminished, reality is concrete and experiential. Therefore, worship leaders most effectively communicate theological concepts in tangible ways.

A recent service focused on images of God. We asked, "When you think of God, what images come to mind?" Among the metaphors mentioned were "judge," "king," "father," and "shepherd." Many were totally silent and even appeared bewildered by the question, reminding us that some had forgotten the word "God."

We affirmed that the Bible has many images for God in addition to those mentioned by the worshipers. This passage from Hosea was read:

Yet it was I who taught Ephraim to walk.
I took them up in my arms;
but they did not know that I healed them.
I led them with cords of human kindness,
with bands of love.
I was to them like those
who lift infants to their cheeks.
I bent down to them and fed them. (11.3–4)

I cradled a soft cuddly doll in my arms as I spoke. I looked into its eyes, and gently stroked its soft face. "Have you ever pictured God as a dad or mom cuddling a baby?" I asked. "That's how Hosea wanted the people to know God," I added.

Then the doll was passed among the worshipers and each was invited to hold it. Everyone eagerly and tenderly cuddled the doll, and the love and caring overflowed. God became visible as worshipers witnessed a neighbor snuggling the doll; and God's love was felt as each nested the baby in his/her bosom. God was no longer an abstract thought or forgotten word, but a lived experience of love made real.

Society tends to assign worth and dignity in relation to our abilities and such qualities as physical appearance, intellectual acumen, productivity, and self-sufficiency. In the early and mid-stages of dementia diseases, people are aware of the decline in their capacity to remember, solve problems, and perform routine tasks. Frequently heard comments are these: "I'm stupid!" "I can't do anything!" "I'm worth nothing!" "I'm losing it!" Or, as one man said repeatedly, "You might as well shoot me!"

How do we help such persons' sense of self-worth and dignity in the context of worship? Accepting and affirming their gifts and participation is one way. Treating them with dignity and worth through touch, smiles, and verbal affirmations is essential. Additionally, the themes and topics around which worship services are constructed counter society's demeaning messages.

A recurring theme of worship at Bethany is assurance that human worth and dignity reside in our identity as beloved sons and daughters of God. A passage used often is 1 John 3.1–2: "See what love the father has for us that we should be called children of God? Beloved, that's who we are. We are God's children now. It does not yet appear what we shall be; but when he appears we shall be like him for we shall see him as he is."

How can such a declaration be concretely illustrated? We have found that the use of an object that belonged to our parents and grandparents is helpful, such as a pocket knife with the handles broken and rusty blades, or a faded and blemished change purse. After showing the knife, for example, the worshipers are asked, "Is this worth anything?" Most will laugh and say, "No!" "But you don't have enough money to buy this from me" was the response.

"Why is this broken, unworkable pocket knife so valuable to me?" I ask. Someone invariably says, "It belonged to your father/grandfather." The message then becomes clear! We are important because of the One to whom we belong! We belong to God! Even if we don't look as we once did or can no longer do what we used to do, we are beloved sons and daughters of God! That gives us infinite worth and dignity.

Or, we might bring a photograph of ourselves as a teenager, show it to the worshipers, and ask, "Who is this?" The resemblance to the person holding the photograph is not immediately evident with the hair loss, wrinkles, sagging skin, and shifting weight. When it becomes clear that the one in the photograph and the one holding it are the same, the appropriate question follows: "Which is more valuable to God?" The point is made!

Although the use of objects appropriate for people in the memory care unit is similar to "children's sermons," the persons present are not children. Treating them as such would further diminish their sense of dignity. The voice tone and demeanor of the leader remains adult interacting with other adults. Otherwise, what the worshiper hears will undermine the message and counter what is seen and/or touched.

Order of worship service at Bethany

Call to Worship and Prayer

Leader: This is the day the Lord has made.
Congregation: Let us rejoice and be glad in it.
Leader: We can sing that now!
Congregation sings:

This is the day, this is the day
That the Lord has made, that the Lord has made.
We will rejoice, we will rejoice,
And be glad in it, and be glad in it.
This is the day that the Lord has made.
We will rejoice and be glad in it.
This is the day, this is the day
That the Lord has made.

Leader: We come together to worship and invite God to be present, hear our praise and our prayers. Let's invite God by singing Kumbayah. What does "kumbayah" mean? (Several respond "Come by here." Congregation sings two verses: "Someone's Singing, Lord" and "Someone's Praying, Lord.")

Prayer of Invocation

Leader: The Lord be with you.
Congregation: And also with you.
Leader: Let us pray.

An extemporaneous prayer is offered, followed by singing "Surely, the Presence of the Lord is in This Place."

Hymn of Praise
Prayers of Thanksgiving

Leader: What are you thankful for today? (Congregants offer expressions of gratitude. After each expression the congregation responds with "Thank you God!")

Doxology

Affirmation of Faith (The affirmation varies each week. Sometimes the Apostles' Creed is used; however, few can recall the words. More often a short Bible verse is repeated as an Affirmation of Faith, such as John 3.16. Psalm 23 is frequently used since most can recite it from memory. The leader may have the congregation repeat after him/her a short verse related to the theme of the day.)

Scripture Reading
Interactive Homily or Reflection on Scripture
Hymn or Chorus Related to Theme

Prayers of Intercession (Congregation is asked "What are your concerns or worries today? Who do you want us to pray for?" Typical responses include family, people who are lonely, the staff, the sick. One worshiper invariably mentions world peace. The leader gathers up the concerns in an extemporaneous prayer.)

The Lord's Prayer (Almost all present join in this prayer from memory.)

Hymn or Chorus ("Blest Be the Tie That Binds" is a popular closing hymn.)

Benediction

Greeting of the People Individually (Each worshiper is greeted by name with a blessing.)

Conclusion

All genuine worship engages the whole person—intellect, feelings, bodily movements, and the senses. We all bring to worship different gifts and varied capacities which enrich the gathered community. Much congregational worship presumes a level of cognitive and language capacities that excludes the growing number of members for whom neuro-cognitive diseases have diminished the ability to participate. Failure to acknowledge the gifts such persons bring to worship relegates them to observers of entertainment or excludes them completely from the worshiping community.

Worship *with* people diagnosed with dementia diseases requires understanding, empathy, compassion, and attentiveness on the part of leaders. In addition, it has been our experience that when warmth of presence and hospitality are extended, those gifts are multiplied and joyfully returned. When we worship *with*, we all experience the God who comes especially among and through the vulnerable, frail, and forgotten, those whom Jesus calls "the least of these."

Things Remembered

Joining Persons with Dementia in the Distinct Beauty of Their Worship

Chaplain Drew DeCrease (Roman Catholic Deacon)

As a hospice chaplain, my goal in providing emotional and spiritual support to persons in their late-life journey is not to beckon them to join me in my walk or my agenda, but rather that I may join *them*—to discover and embrace the sacredness of their journey and the forms of worship unique to them at this time in their lives and at this stage of their physical and cognitive health.

Perhaps half of those I visit and with whom I worship are persons who have dementia. Little did I know when I began working in this role five years ago that they would make possible the most enriching and beautiful worship experiences of my life. We say prayers, we sing hymns, and we share the ways that God has touched our lives...but not necessarily in conventional times, or places, or ways.

Amongst caregivers, I've heard it wisely said, "If you've seen one person with dementia, you've seen...one person with dementia." Understanding this uniqueness is key for those who would facilitate worship. One dear woman I visited for years (I'll call her Mary Lou) had a limited vocabulary, which gradually diminished to the point at which she was no longer able to speak at all. She and her husband were devout Christians, and when I accompanied him to visit Mary Lou, we often sang her favorite hymns to her. Her way of participating in worship was to tap her feet. As we would lead off with "In the Garden" or "The Old Rugged Cross," Mary Lou would smile, and we would see her feet begin to tap. Something so simple—tapping one's feet to music—meant the world to Mary Lou's husband, because it communicated to him that his wife of 63 years was still "with us," enjoying his presence as her loving husband, and enjoying the presence of the Lord by joining in worship, in the manner still possible for her.

When I first began my role of hospice chaplain, I attended a service in a dementia unit which taught me volumes. It was a blessing/spiritual healing service led by an Anglican deacon. I perceived immediately the challenge she faced as a worship leader, because the congregation of 20, gathered in an activities area, was primarily persons with severe physical and cognitive disabilities. Some appeared to be sleeping or non-responsive. Some I knew to have hearing loss. The deacon asked me to accompany her, as she made her way from person to person. Upon each person's head, she placed her hands (and invited me to put my hand lightly on their shoulder). Speaking close to the ear of each person, she prayed for God's love to be poured out on them, God's presence felt, God's peace descending. For me, it was an intense and humbling experience, as I saw one after another apparently non-responsive person respond with a deep and gentle joy—uttering a "Thank you," or squeezing her hand, crying a few tears, beaming with a smile. I learned that day that worship for dementia patients need not be diminished in scope or intensity, and may, on the contrary, be a profoundly spiritual experience.

There are many things forgotten by persons with dementia; what is often a surprise and a joy to me, however, is that there are also many things remembered. As a lifetime player of stringed instruments, I often carry a guitar or banjo with me when I visit, and I incorporate music into all of my worship services. When dementia has taken away much of a person's ability to communicate verbally, music often unlocks the door of speech which has appeared to be closed, or nearly closed. The little miracle that I witness regularly is this: a person who is barely speaking, or is confused in their speech, is able to sing every word of "Jesus Loves Me" or another well-known hymn. Many times I have listened in amazement as words which cannot be spoken…are *sung*.

That which has been most repeated in one's life is most likely to be remembered by a person with dementia. After a lifetime of saying the Lords' Prayer…when other words no longer flow, these words often do. A best-loved prayer, like a best-loved hymn, can also open the door to further speech—the prayer or the song prompting verbalization beyond what seemed possible. Experiencing this in persons with dementia calls to my mind the words of the prophet Ezekiel: "…but when I speak with you, I will loosen your tongue…" (Ezekiel 3.27; *New English Translation* (*NET*)).

In the setting of worship with persons who have dementia, I often take the approach of naming popular hymns, attempting to discern which hymns are best known by the particular group I am with. This makes for a less structured service, but one which is more effective in inviting participation. My advice is to come prepared with music for the classic, best-loved hymns, and then let the Spirit, and the congregation, lead. Joining *their* journey, you will take rich spiritual paths that may have otherwise remained untrodden in your life!

Another "teachable moment" for me was when I attended a worship service for persons with dementia led by a pastor who was a particularly good storyteller. She chose a children's story that celebrated the beauty and wonder of the universe, the handiwork of the Creator. The language was basic, but the spiritual concepts were soaring. A story told engagingly is a marvelous way to connect with persons with dementia, and perhaps the most effective way to prompt dialogue. I was asked to bring my guitar and be ready to play "He's Got the Whole World in His Hands" to complement the story. As the song was known to all since their early childhood, the participation was robust, smiles all around, and a deeply comforting feeling that God did indeed have "you and me brother, you and me sister, in His hands."

As I began to lead worship services for persons with dementia on my own, I once centered a service on the images evoked in the hymn "How Great Thou Art." I invited the attendees to "Consider all the works thy hand has made," and we talked about "the stars, the rolling thunder, the woods, the forest glades, the birds singing sweetly in the trees, the mountains, the brooks, the gentle breeze." To enhance the worship experience, I included in a hand-out an image of each: one photo of a winding brook, one of a bluebird singing, one of a lush forest... This provided the opportunity to talk about the experience of God in Creation, and to revel in what has been given to us by God's hand. The images facilitated participation and discussion; even those who could not verbalize were engaged as they looked at the beautiful photos (which they were invited to keep, for reflection through the day). I realized that I had stumbled upon something important—that visuals enhance the ability of persons with dementia to join into worship. I try always to bring images with me to hand out at these services, with a few key words on the sheet for spiritual reflection.

Yes, much has been forgotten by persons with dementia, but there are also many things remembered; and those are often things central to the Good News of the Scriptures and to the heart of God. When we bring our spiritual focus to the core and center of our own faith, clear and unencumbered, we are ready to join in their spiritual journey.

Worship Brainstorming

Robin Dill (Nondenominational Christian)

In my position as Director of Grace Arbor, a congregational Respite Program of First United Methodist Church, one of the activities I regularly do with our participants and volunteers is brainstorm a topic. This delightful activity can be used to generate games and gifts, as well as get our folks' brains stimulated by making connections to thoughts and memories they hadn't considered in a while. Brainstorming leads to "rabbit trails" which lead to more connections! To get started I will write a topic or just a word on the white board and ask them, "What does this word make you think of?" or "What comes to mind when you hear the word…?" I will ask this question several times in many ways as we talk about it. If a story bubbles up, I will give the invitation to "tell us about it."

One week, in preparation for conversations about this book on worship resources for clergy, I decided to explore the word *worship* with our folks. I did this at the beginning of our devotional time. I told them that I was part of a project that had to do with worship and I wanted them to tell me what came to mind when they heard the word "worship." After this first session I left their responses up on the white board and we added to our list over the entire week. We spent a few minutes each day adding to the list. These sessions prompted stories and significant memories about worship experiences. One lady told of how her dad always sung to her the hymn "What a Friend We Have in Jesus." Since this brainstorming experience, we sing that hymn frequently because of her response and the joy she feels singing it. Another idea I had was to invite the staff of the church our ministry is a part of to share their favorite prayers from the Bible and tell us why they loved them. I created a week's worth of devotions from that one idea!

Of all the activities we do, our devotion time is the most poignant. From singing hymns to opening up the scriptures together, the responses from our participants are different than those from nonspiritual activities. These moments bring back memories where stories are told about teaching children's church, or military experiences where people were told to hide Bibles due to the country they were in. When we explored the word worship, just hearing the lady, who wasn't communicating well on any level, share about her dad singing to her as a child was so valuable. Often, I will try to capture these moments in my journal to be shared at a later date with their caregivers.

As you read through the following list we created together, imagine what words you might use to brainstorm with a group of people with dementia. You will be inspired to do this activity again, I'm sure! Take time to be present, fully, as you do this activity. Be spontaneous and see what emerges. Be prepared to be blessed, as well!

Worship

- Go to church
- Pray
- Praise
- Adoration
- Thanksgiving
- God
- Calm
- Gratitude
- Group of people
- One step up from a door
- Friendship
- Honor
- Communication with God
- Honoring God
- My dad
- Happiness
- Forgiveness
- Sitting up in the mountains taking in His wondrous works

- Prayer
- Music
- Listening
- Peace
- Love
- Love of God
- Tithes and offerings
- The Lord
- Thankfulness to God
- Relationship with God
- Our future
- Jesus
- Unity
- Worship in the way—sincere
- Loving and kind—tell people who need to hear in this way
- Group of people worshiping
- Trust
- God filling our minds and our hearts—we then respond
- Singing

Devotions in the Respite Care Setting

Robin Dill (Nondenominational Christian)

For the past 12 years I have directed a congregational respite ministry for adults with dementia. The term “respite” means a “time-out.” Respite ministry is literally a time-out for caregivers while their loved ones participate in the activities our ministry offers. This ministry is housed in First United Methodist Church of Lawrenceville, Georgia. Grace Arbor, the name of our ministry, meets four days per week for five hours each day. We have an average of 12–15 participants and 10 volunteers each day. Daily we have set aside a time of worship, which we simply call “Devotions.” It lasts about 45 minutes to an hour, and our format is like a mini-worship experience that is highly interactive. The components of our devotion time are: an opening prayer, hymn singing, use of devotional booklets, more hymn singing, and a closing prayer.

Opening prayer

We begin our devotional time with a short prayer. It is a way to settle us down and prepare us for the time ahead. It may sound like:

> Heavenly Father, we thank You for this day. We thank You for the blessing of being Your children and ask that You would meet us in this time of devotions. Bless us with Your presence and open our hearts to what You want us to receive. In Jesus’ Name we pray, Amen.

Hymn singing

We spend about 15–20 minutes singing hymns. (We use the book *Hymns We Love to Sing*. This is a large print, spiral bound book with words only.[2]) I might choose hymns related to the topic of our devotional booklet for that day or ask for suggestions from our participants or volunteers.

---

2 Whitmore, A. (1995) *Hymns We Love to Sing*. Kelowna, BC, Canada: Woodlake Publishing.

Devotional booklets

In 2007 I completed a Montessori for Dementia training. A component of the training was called Reading Roundup. A group of people would gather together to learn about a topic using printed booklets. I took this idea and created our devotional booklets. Each booklet has cover art, questions to arouse interest in the topic, scriptural text and reflection questions, closing statements, and application thoughts. Each person gets their own booklet or can share with the person sitting next to them. The booklets are printed in an Arial font of 18 count or larger with left-hand double staples. Page numbers are included in a larger bold font on the right-hand corner. Pages can be one- or two-sided. I keep each group of devotions in a manila folder with the title on it. (I have three filing cabinets filled with devotional booklets! They can be used year after year or repeated as needed.)[3] These booklets are designed to be interactive. I begin with the cover...

Discussion surrounding the cover

The "cover art" pertains to the devotion for that day. This may include a photo, a piece of art, or even clip art. Often I will begin this discussion with: "I wonder why this particular photo or art was chosen for this topic." This cover will be in color so that even the colors can be explored. If you are familiar with the MoMA (Museum of Modern Art) Alzheimer's Project, the cover art can be a mini-project.[4] We may take five minutes or more to explore the cover, with me asking questions like: "What is happening in the picture? How does the picture make you feel? What is

---

3 Conducting daily devotionals over these past 12 years at Grace Arbor, I have written several series of devotionals, as well as many individual devotions. I have saved many of them on CDs and they are available to anyone who would find them helpful. Some examples are:

- I Corinthians 13, The Love Chapter (15 devotions)
- The Fruit of the Spirit (11 devotions)
- The Psalms (17 devotions)
- Lent to Easter and Beyond (9 devotions)
- Advent to Epiphany (9 devotions)
- Playing by the Rules (10 devotions)

Please do not hesitate to contact me: Robin Dill, robin.dill@comcast.net

4 The MoMA Alzheimer's Project is an ongoing interactive art experience for people with dementia and their caregivers that originated in New York City and has now spread to museums all over the United States.

the setting of the picture?" Questions like these can make the experience rich and help prepare the participants for what is inside the booklet.

Opening comments and questions

These comments and questions "set up" the scripture we will explore. The purpose is to get the participants' brains stimulated and their hearts engaged. Some of my comments or prompts may include background information about the scripture we will be exploring. For example, in my "Epiphany" booklet, I will begin by saying:

> "Epiphany…hmmm…wonder what this word means? Any ideas? Share. Have you ever had an epiphany?"
>
> "Today we are going to talk about gifts and the people who brought gifts to baby Jesus. We think of January 6th as Epiphany. It is the date celebrated in the Christian church that the wise men brought gifts to Jesus."

Then I will ask some questions about gifts and take the time to listen to the responses:

> "What is a gift?"
>
> "What is a gift that you have a memory of as a child?"
>
> "What is a gift that you have a memory of as an adult?"
>
> "What makes something a gift?"

The next part is the scriptural text. Depending on the scripture, I will choose a certain translation. The text will be referenced (in this example I have cited Matthew 2.1–12, *New International Version*).

After we read the text we will follow up with application/relevancy questions. They may include references to the actual scripture: "What is speaking to your heart as you read the scripture?"—or questions that relate to the scripture: "You are seven years old. You have been asked to be in an Epiphany play and you will play the part of one of the wise men. What gift will you bring to baby Jesus?" "You are now 15 years old and have been asked to be in an Epiphany play as one of the wise men. What gift will you bring to baby Jesus?" "You are now present-day age and have been asked to be in an Epiphany play as one of the wise men. What gift will you bring to baby Jesus?"

Closing prayer and/or one more hymn

Depending on time constraints and the attention span of the participants, we will sing one more hymn or just close with a short prayer. I invite everyone to hold the person's hand on either side of them. Our closing prayer may be as simple as something like this:

> "Thank You Father God for the gift of Your Son, Jesus Christ. Help us to share the gift of His love with all we meet. Amen."

Or, we might pray the Lord's Prayer together.

That All May Worship

Creative Worship for Persons with Dementia

Rev. Dr. Richard L. Morgan (Presbyterian Church, USA) and Rev. David J. Fetterman (United Methodist)

Helpful elements in ordering a worship service

The following elements are helpful in ordering weekly worship services for persons with dementia:

- Familiar music
- Memory cues
- Visual and tactile symbols with music
- The sacrament of the Lord's Supper
- Closing affirmation.

Familiar music

There is a saying among those of us who work with persons with dementia: "Music is the last thing to go." Some of our earliest experiences of God occur in childhood. We associate these experiences with hymns that were popular in our churches at that time. Music has the power to evoke memories. Helen was 86 years old and suffering from Alzheimer's disease. She rarely spoke. Her short-term memory was around 30 seconds. While we were singing "Blessed Assurance," she began to move her lips and then sing, clearly articulating the words. Caregivers were astonished to hear her sing. Apparently the music had reached beyond the dementia to her soul.

Music influences the motor center of the brain that responds directly to auditory rhythmic cues and does not require cognitive functioning. It allows caregivers and care receivers to connect with one another. Scripture records how the sweet songs of David became therapeutic for the dark moods and depression of King Saul, as in this passage from I Samuel:

> Whenever the evil spirit from God affected Saul, David would take the lyre and play it. Then Saul would relax and feel better, and the evil spirit would leave him alone. (16.23, *Common English Bible*)

On several occasions David's songs lifted Saul's soul from depression when his mind was tormented by the burdens of being king of Israel.

Any kind of music can break down the walls of cognitive failure that hinder persons with dementia. Jack, in the last stages of dementia, sat listlessly in his room at the end of the hall. His daughter had brought his old record player to the room, hoping he would listen to some of his old records. She played some of Benny Goodman's music. When Jack heard the music of the clarinet and horn, he began to keep time with the music, tapping his feet to the tune and even singing the melody of the song. Music lifted Jack from his lethargy and enabled him to experience a measure of happiness in the moment.

Memory cues

In general, persons with dementia are intellectually impaired and may not be able to understand words or express themselves. However, certain memory cues can facilitate their understanding. The sign of the cross, a crucifix, or other visual objects remind them of their faith.

Well-known and beloved scriptures and prayer, such as the 23rd Psalm and the Lord's Prayer, seem to get through to persons with dementia. They probably memorized these words in childhood, hid them in their souls, and may even be able to speak some of the words. The use of uplifted hands in blessing and passing the peace are other ways to express faith beyond words. Sometimes, if you are ordained, wearing a stole reminds them of their religious leader. It is amazing how persistent the memory for things said, done, or worn can be over a lifetime.

Dick (Richard Morgan): A friend of mine made a wooden cross with the Greek letters Alpha and Omega carved on it. I placed the cross on the piano before every worship service. In one service Jean asked, "I see the cross, but what are those strange letters on the cross?" I explained that they are the Alpha and Omega, meaning that Christ is the first and the last and that he is with us at the beginning of life and at its end. She seemed to understand.

Visual and tactile symbols with music

Being able to associate an object they can see or touch with old hymns becomes a powerful form of worship for people with dementia. Some effective ways to use music and symbols in worship include:

- Sing "Turn Your Eyes Upon Jesus" at every worship service. As you sing, point to a picture of Jesus. Another possibility is to hold up Heinrich Hofmann's picture of Jesus in Gethsemane which can still be found in many churches. Residents may associate these things with their childhood churches.

Dick: Sometimes I actually move to one side of the room with the picture, and motion to the residents to turn their eyes toward the picture as we sing the first phrase, "Turn your eyes upon Jesus, look full in his wonderful face." Once I told the story of Peter walking on the water, emphasizing that as long as he kept his eyes on Jesus, he did not sink in the waves of the storm.

- "The Church in the Wildwood" ("There's a church in the valley by the wildwood") is another song from their childhood that they love to sing. Someone built a little brown wooden church with white shutters, a white door, and a steeple. The little church is shown to the group and then passed from person to person. Some of the residents finger the cross on the door or on the windows.

  When you sing the line "No spot is so dear to my childhood as the little brown church in the vale," pause and ask individuals, "Tell me about your church." Often they will begin talking about their childhood church, for that is where many of them are in the present moment. During one of these discussions one woman became distraught and said, "I forgot to bring my Bible today," just as she actually did going to her church of long ago.

- Another favorite hymn from the past is "Rock of Ages, Cleft for Me." Sing the first stanza and stop. Show them small rocks that are large enough to be held in a hand. Pass the rocks from row to row. As they touch the rocks you will have no idea of what they sense; but you will have offered another sensory experience into the worship through this tactile activity. Then sing "Rock of Ages, cleft for me, let me hide myself in thee," once again telling them that often people of God hid behind rocks for shelter and safety. Not all will understand, but some will.

- When you sing "In the Garden," a perennial favorite, direct their attention to the garden outside if there is one, or bring a few plants and flowers to show to them. Perhaps you can consider having some roses to show as you sing the line "I come to the garden alone while the dew is still on the roses." Look into their eyes when you sing "And he walks with me, and he talks with me, and he tells me I am his own," and sense God's presence in these people's hearts as they relive this song of their childhood.

Dick: I walked over to one woman who was nearing the end of her life. I sang the words to her, and she reached out with her bony hands and grasped me. Surely God did walk with her and talk with her in a way I cannot understand.

- In the autumn sing "This Is My Father's World." Read Psalm 1 and show a large poster of the words of Ecclesiastes 3.1: "For every thing there is a season and a time for every matter under heaven." Show the worshipers different colors of leaves, symbolizing the changing seasons—green leaves, bright red leaves, and brown leaves—and suggest how the seasons of life change, and yet each one displays the glory of God.

  Here are some more suggestions for worshiping through music and symbols:

  - Show a picture of a sparrow and sing "His Eye Is on the Sparrow."
  - Display a picture of Jesus blessing the children and sing "Jesus Loves Me."
  - Wear dark glasses and then regular glasses as you sing "Open My Eyes That I May See."
  - Show a cross and sing "The Old Rugged Cross."
  - Take a piece of string and place it around the group as you sing "Blest Be the Tie That Binds."

- Use a carving or photo of an old sea captain or a lighthouse and sing "Love Lifted Me," or "Let the Lower Lights Be Burning."
- Show the group rosary beads and a clock. Then sing "Take Time to Be Holy."
- Display a large Bible and sing "The B-i-b-l-e."
- Light a small candle and sing "This Little Light of Mine."
- Make a sign or poster of Psalm 119.105 (*King James Version*): "Thy Word is a lamp unto my feet, and a light unto my path." Shine a flashlight on the floor, and then walk a few steps as you explain that the Bible shows us where we are and lights our path so we know where to go.

Dick: One of the favorite choruses we sing at the end of worship is "You Are Mine" by David Haas.

> Do not be afraid, I am with you.
>
> I have called you each by name,
>
> Come and follow me,
>
> I will bring you home.
>
> I love you and you are mine.[5]

When we come to the line "I have called you each by name," the pianist pauses while I go around the room and say each person's name. I can't understand it, but the words of this chorus seem to reach each person's spirit.

Anyone who leads worship for persons with dementia needs to be creative and intentional about speaking to their hearts and souls when their cognitive functioning is either deficient or absent.

5 Text copyright © 1991 by GIA Publications, Inc.; 7404 S. Mason Ave., Chicago, IL 60638; www.giamusic.com; or 800-442-1358. All rights reserved. Used by permission.

The sacrament of the Lord's Supper

Some clergy will not give Holy Communion to persons with dementia. They believe these persons do not comprehend the meaning of the sacrament and have no idea of what they are doing. Refusing to give them Communion denies the gospel and meaning of the sacrament. The sacrament does not depend on us understanding it. How can we, regardless of our cognition, understand the depths and breadth of God's grace embedded in the Eucharist? The sacrament does not depend on us but on God. God offers grace unconditionally to all who receive it.

The sacrament is a mystery. Life is best defined not by rational intelligence but by mystery. The mystery does not require our understanding but our participation with wonder at God's grace. That sense of wonder in the Lord's Supper is available to all persons, including those with dementia.

In addition, memory is not simply the mental recollection of the sacrament but also a lived connection with the past. Individuals with dementia may not recall when or where they took the sacrament in their past, but they sense God's presence through receiving the sacrament. To deny them the sacrament is to deprive them of the most important Presence available to them.

Careful preparation needs to be made in offering this sacrament to persons with dementia. We must be sure the residents do not choke when they swallow the bread. Use small pieces of bread or wafers. It is wise to always have a glass of water available. The sacrament should be given to each person individually, saying their name, as you say, "This is Christ's body, broken for you."

Dave (David Fetterman): I was a chaplain in a memory care unit where we celebrated the Eucharist on a monthly basis. Residents would sit around a long table. Many of them were in advanced stages of Alzheimer's disease or a related dementia. Communication was usually non-verbal. As I went from person to person with the broken bread, they would raise their hands cupping them in anticipation of me placing a piece of bread there—just as they had probably done many times before. Much had left their memories but not the meaning of this sacrament.

Closing affirmation

What's in a name?

The short answer to that question is "a lot." There is a lot in a name. It conveys identity. Parents often spend lots of time selecting names for their children. One of their objectives is often to select a name that conveys something special about the child to be named. In some faiths names are given at or after baptism to connote the new life signified in this sacrament. In Genesis, Jacob's name is changed to Israel to connote a change brought about due to a faith encounter with God (Genesis 32.28). Names convey special identity and are important.

Names also portray uniqueness. They provide a way to separate one person from another. Can you imagine an elementary classroom where all of the students had the same name? What a nightmare for the teacher! Beyond separating one person from another, names convey that we are special. We aren't called "Person A" or "Child B" or the like. We are called "David," "Dick," "Pat," "Alice Ann," and so forth. We are special, unique. Our names help to indicate that to all the world. Knowing the names of the individuals in our care in Memory units is important to reminding people that they are special, unique children of God. Having names is important. Knowing them is critical for compassionate care.

The importance of touch

A reading of the Gospels reveals how important the sense of touch was to Jesus. Scripture records many instances of Jesus touching people and of people trying to touch him. When Jesus touched the lepers, the blind, and the woman who touched the hem of his garment, healing and power were present in his touch. For many of the persons in our care, touch is seldom experienced. To hold a hand while praying or to gently touch a shoulder during an encounter can help the person to feel alive and loved, while a resistance to offer appropriate touches can lead to feelings of isolation and unworthiness. For example, it can be such an important and simple act of caring to go around the group before worship, touching hands and welcoming each person by name. Going around the group at the end of the service, again touching hands, and offering a blessing by name can be a powerful and loving way to conclude a worship experience. We need to be aware of God's presence as we touch each person. Some of their responses are verbal, like "Thank you," or "God bless you." Touch somehow evokes some kind of healing in the person as well as an important human connection—important things for those in danger of spiritual and emotional isolation.

Dick: My wife, Alice Ann, and I always have a closing ritual with those who attend worship. At times we pass the peace and move around the room to look at each person. We grasp their hands and say, "The peace of God be with you." Usually they respond in kind or smile. We hug when they seem receptive or place our hands on their shoulders.

Expect the unexpected

Dick: In a nursing home where I served as a chaplain, a guest minister's sermon was much too long for the residents. When he finally finished he said, "I have really enjoyed being here. I would love to come back." One woman replied in a loud voice, "I sure hope not!"

Here is one word of counsel for anyone leading worship for persons with dementia: expect the unexpected. Anything can happen.

Some individuals will blurt out words that could disrupt the service—comments like "Oh shut up!" or "I have to go to the toilet," or "It's too hot in here."

Dick: Once during Communion a distraught woman took the bread in her hand. She squeezed it and then dropped the crumbs on the floor. She was embarrassed, but I gently put another piece of bread in her mouth, and she was happy. We must give more than crumbs to people with dementia. They need the living bread of God, revealed in Jesus Christ. His broken body provides health and peace for their broken minds.

Dr. Dwyn Mounger tells the story of someone with Alzheimer's who wandered into a chapel in a nursing home where he was giving Communion. Before anyone could stop her, the confused and bewildered woman rushed to the holy table and, with one sweep of her arms, knocked off the tray of Communion wine. There was a sickening noise as it hit the floor, and the tiny glasses fell out, spilling the wine into a great stream as it spread across the floor. Some attending the service gasped, while others displayed no concern.

If something like this happened at a service you were leading, you could tell the residents that this accident was a symbol of the death of Jesus. The spilled wine was a symbol of Christ's blood, given for us.

At one service, a man named Ralph, who had been a circuit judge, now had severe dementia. He came to worship in a Geri-Chair and was usually quiet and composed. In the midst of singing "Rock of Ages, Cleft for Me," he began pounding his chair and shouting, "Let the court come to order. Let the court come to order." For one shining moment he was back in his courtroom, in charge of the proceedings, and so proud of his control. Dick walked slowly to Ralph's chair, clasped his hand, and said, "Judge, the court is in order. Let the proceedings begin." He quieted down, and worship proceeded.

Ray Inscoe, former director of pastoral care at Westminster Canterbury, a retirement community in Richmond, Virginia, shared a profound story from his experience. A resident who moved into the community told him she had lost her faith and had become an atheist. She developed dementia and entered personal care. Ray noticed that she began to attend weekly Bible study and worship, where she demonstrated a vibrant faith. Her dementia caused her to forget her doubts and unbelief and to return to the foundation of her childhood faith.

Dave: I usually keep my eyes slightly open during prayer in a memory care unit—and this is why. When I first began as a chaplain, our facility conducted worship in the activities room of our memory care unit. Beside the area for worship was a small kitchen where the residents had cooking activities. Howard would often roll over to the stove in his wheelchair and try to lift the stove top. From what began as an unexpected event the first time he did it, I learned to keep praying aloud, walk over to Howard, and gently redirect him to a safer place—all without skipping a beat.

Mutual spiritual practice

Sometimes the effort required to read scripture, pray together, or attend a service is just too much for individuals with dementia. This is especially true in the middle and later stages of the disease, when the person is increasingly confused and confined to the home or nursing home.

When this happens, there seem to be few options for mutual worship or spiritual practice. At times when the person seems lucid, try some of the following activities, which will also benefit you as the caregiver:

- Listen together to a recording of well-known and well-loved hymns.
- For Catholics: say the rosary together. Many people whose dementia is far advanced can still remember the words to the Hail Mary and watch Mass on television.
- Keep the Christmas manger scene on display all year. Stamped in our earliest memories, these figures bring consolation.
- Borrow some children's Bible story books with lots of large pictures. Persons with dementia can still relate to simple pictures long after they can no longer understand or follow TV or movies.
- When the person you are caring for is silent and still, take time to rest during that moment in God. Practice deep breathing and imagine you are breathing in the comforting Spirit of God each time you inhale. When you exhale, imagine yourself breathing out the peace and love of God into the air surrounding your loved one.
- Watch videos of nature scenes. They are usually accompanied by hymns or other lovely music. These videos have no plot and they don't demand an intellectual response, as would a TV program, so they are likely to be enjoyed far into the dementing process.

A challenge

Dick reflected on the future once:

> One morning as I reflected on the worship service while sauntering down to my apartment on "the other side," I had these thoughts: *In 20 years, unless a cure is found, millions of baby boomers will have Alzheimer's or some form of dementia. If they are residents in care facilities, what hymns will they sing? Will they still sing the old hymns? Or will they sing more contemporary hymns like "Lord of the Dance," "Here I Am Lord," and "God of the Sparrow, God of the Whale"? Or will they sing praise choruses?* Then I remembered an old hymn I learned as a child, "Tell Me the Old, Old Story." Remembering those precious people in that memory care place, some of the words took on new meaning.

Tell me the old, old story
Of unseen things above
Of Jesus and his glory,
Of Jesus and his love.
Tell me the story simply,
As to a little child.

Tell me the story slowly,
That I may take it in,

tell me the story often,
for I forget so soon;

tell me the old, old story:
"Christ Jesus makes thee whole."

("Tell Me the Old, Old Story," Katherine Hankey 1834–1911)

We who are charged with leading worship with those with Alzheimer's disease and related dementias would do well to heed Dick in this. We are living in a changing world. In it people have changing views and connections with the religious resources that many of us have held near and dear over the years.

How do we tell the "old, old story" in ways that new ears will be able to find comfort and meaning as their memories fade? First, we can cherish the old, old stories that form the core of our faith traditions. Second, we can make a point of learning what rituals and spiritual resources are infusing new generations with meaning. Third, we can know those with whom we come into contact well—their culture, generation, and background. Fourth, we can begin to integrate what we have learned about evolving spiritual resources into services with participants of newer generations.

For Christians, a beauty of the gospel message is its timelessness: its ability to remain fresh and relevant as the times in which it is told change. Other religious traditions can stay the same within their contexts. May we accept the challenge to "tell the old, old story" with new generations in fresh ways, always seeking ways to provide them with triggers to memory that provide meaning and hope.

Note: Adapted from Jane Marie Thibault and Richard L. Morgan, *No Act of Love is Ever Wasted*. Copyright 2009. Used with permission of Upper Room Publishing, 1908 Grand Ave., Nashville, TN 37212.

Sensing the Sacred

A Small Group Worship Experience for Those with Alzheimer's and Other Dementias

Rev. Nancy Gordon (Lutheran)

I came to working with older adults after attending seminary in mid-life and then serving for five years as an associate pastor of a congregation. I had no real experience working with older adults and I accepted a challenge when Friendship Village of Schaumburg, IL, a large retirement community, hired me to oversee all the resident programming, including chaplaincy. Recognizing my need for education in this field, my immediate supervisor suggested that I participate in the Geriatric Pastoral Care Institute located at Luther Seminary. Thus, I found myself in St. Paul, MN, for two weeks in the summers of 1998 and 1999. That experience was invaluable as I jumped into developing the Growth Opportunities Program for Friendship Village. In that process, I found that working with older adults was a privilege and decided to provide the best possible care and programming.

I quickly discovered that the traditional, word-oriented worship service that we were providing just did not work with persons with Alzheimer's. It was evident that the music and the scripture readings often reached them, but the traditional sermon (even if it was very short) did not.

Building on *Young Children and Worship*

I remembered a worship program designed for children that used wooden figures as a way to visually tell a story from scripture. I knew women from my congregation who had been trained in telling these stories and bringing this worship to the children of our congregation. They found learning and presenting the stories was beneficial to their own spiritual lives, as well as being an effective way for children to experience the biblical story.

I had some concerns about using a children's program with older adults. It was important to me to be respectful of the years they had experienced and I didn't want them to feel that they were being talked down to in any way. But I was encouraged to try using this program with the residents because I had been the recipient of these stories when I attended a pastor's retreat. Sonja Stewart, who developed the program and co-authored the book *Young Children and Worship* (Stewart and Berryman 1989), was the storyteller to the pastors at this retreat, and I found that receiving the stories in this way was moving and soul stirring. I didn't feel talked down to at all.

While considering whether to use this program, I was at the same time learning about Alzheimer's disease and what happens to persons who are experiencing the disease. I realized that the adults I was serving in the dementia care area had lost a lot of the ability to process language—both in hearing and speaking. It was also evident that talking to them in conceptual and abstract ways did not work at all.

I was also learning that even with their difficulties with language processing and understanding abstract concepts, along with their memory issues, persons with dementia were not that different from anyone else. They were persons who lived in relationship with others and who continued to seek meaning in their lives. Serving them was an opportunity to join them in their present moment and to focus on the experience of that moment. They were also persons who had the ability to continue to take action and they were spiritual beings. It was incumbent upon us to find a way to meet them where they were and to support their spiritual journeys even at this stage of their lives.

The article "Actions, feelings, and values: Foundations of meaning and personhood in dementia" suggests that persons with dementia are still making choices in the living of their lives and "can still be held accountable for loving God and fellow human beings" (McFadden, Ingram, and Olson Baldauf 2001, p.82). Hanson, Mabry, and Williams (2003) reflected on the need for spiritual companions and spiritual nourishment for persons suffering with dementia. The authors suggested that the need for spiritual nourishment could be met by providing a safe place for feelings, and for comfort and reassurance along with rituals and stories that linked them to their spiritual history and traditions.

The *Young Children and Worship* program provided a worship structure that could be that safe place and the rituals and stories that would be remembered by those in the Christian tradition. The structure and methodology of the service not only grew out of Christian tradition, but was designed using concepts that Maria Montessori developed in working with children. Montessori developed segmented, small group activities to help children learn, build self-esteem, and focus on a task. Montessori learning is based on the manipulation of objects. Thus, it is more demonstration based and oriented to the physical, rather than abstract concepts and speech. Montessori-based activities support a sense of self-worth, give residents opportunities to express thoughts and feelings, give them the opportunity to be part of a group, and provide a sense of accomplishment and success as well as a sense of order and safety (Keane and Ustick 2003).

While working at the retirement community and wondering if this program could be adapted for use with older adults with Alzheimer's and other dementias of aging, I applied for a Vital Worship Grant from the Calvin Institute of Christian Worship (located on the campus of Calvin College, Grand Rapids, MI) for the purpose of developing the program and piloting it. The grant I received enabled me to go to a week-long training with Sonja Stewart at Western Theological Seminary in Holland, MI. There I learned about the children's program, its whys and wherefores, and how to do it from the originator herself. She later came to Friendship Village to help in a training session with volunteers.

Stewart stressed that the program needed to be presented in the way it was designed. There were both theological and Montessori concepts behind each part of it and she was adamant that it not be changed. She was also adamant that this was a worship service and the leader needed to be prepared by knowing the story so it could be told and figures moved in the most efficient way possible. She noted that this takes practice! And she emphasized that the presenter/storyteller must be spiritually prepared for telling the story. In the older adult realm this means that this is not just an activity that anyone can lead, but it is a Christian worship service and must be led by a person (not necessarily a pastor) who has both the faith and the gifts to lead a service of worship.

The worship service

As I worked on developing the program I named it *Sensing the Sacred* to stress that it was a sensory approach to worship, rather than a conceptual approach. The *Sensing the Sacred* worship service is a ritual of worship for six to eight people that follows very closely the *Young Children and Worship* order of service. As it was for the children, this service is a time to experience and to praise God. It meets the needs of the participants for God and a religious community, as well as the needs for love, security, continuity, order, and meaning. The approach to worship is primarily visual, oral, and kinesthetic. The service is structured and done the same way every time.

Order of worship

1. Assemble in God's Name
    - i. Call to worship
    - ii. The greeting
    - iii. Songs of praise
    - iv. Preparing to hear a story of God
2. Proclaim God's Word
    - i. Telling the story
    - ii. Responding by wondering together and reading the story from scripture
3. Give Thanks to God
    - i. Giving thanks by singing
    - ii. Giving thanks by naming someone or something we're thankful for
    - iii. Giving thanks by praying (leader prays, including spoken thanksgivings, and then ends the prayer with the Lord's Prayer)
4. Go in God's Name
    - i. Singing a hymn
    - ii. Benediction by leader
    - iii. Personal word of blessing to each participant by name

I left out two areas of the worship service as designed by Stewart in response to the story, which were a "feast" and an art opportunity. The chaplains and I tried including them when we first piloted the program but it proved to make the whole experience too long and complicated for the presenters and the participants.

The goals of this worship

Creation of sacred space and time

The average skilled nursing facility (SNF) does not have a designated chapel, so the space available for religious services usually doubles as the dining room or activity room. My team and I found, however, that sacred space and time were created by the structure of the service, the simple and three-dimensional storytelling, singing hymns, reading scripture, listening to one of God's stories, and extending and receiving God's blessing.

Experiencing God

The storytelling is done with an economy of words and motion, where the teller is looking at the story ground and figures, *not at the participants.* This focused attention on the story figures is done so that the story itself, not the storyteller, is the focus of attention.

This was a point of discussion when I was considering the program. Other chaplains told me that it wouldn't work because it was impossible to do a presentation with those with Alzheimer's without maintaining eye contact with the members of the group. They believed that the attention of the group was kept through eye contact. I decided to try it as Sonja Stewart recommended by presenting with my eyes on the figures at all times in the telling of the story. By keeping my eyes on the story figures, I got out of the way, and participants could experience a meeting with God in the story. I found that while not everyone was always 100 percent attentive, it seemed to be working. I had confirmation that this was so when a housekeeper watching the story from the hallway commented afterwards how the participants were watching and paying attention. She ended with: "That never happens!"

Thus, it's in hearing and seeing a story from God's word that the listeners are invited into the story so they can have an experience of God, rather than simply being told about God. The content of the story itself may soon be lost, but the experience of the Spirit lingers.

Hope in lost places

The experience of dementia is one of loss and feeling lost. As the ability to assimilate, process, and remember old and new information decreases, the world becomes an increasingly chaotic and seemingly unsafe place. Against this backdrop the stories of the Good Shepherd and Jesus and Zacchaeus, the Easter story, and the Advent/Christmas story reiterate God's love, care, and presence. Being known by God by name is a recurring theme in the stories that leads participants to an experience of God's love and care.

How *Sensing the Sacred* can be used

This program is designed to provide a small-group Christian worship experience for those who have been grounded in the Christian tradition. (I developed this in my Christian tradition, but I would encourage those of other faiths to think how it could be used in their context.) It can be delivered by chaplains and/or volunteers in nursing homes and memory care units. It can also be a ministry of congregations who take the program to local elder care residential communities and to members of their church who can no longer attend worship because of age-related dementia. Used in that way it allows members of a family to worship together in a way that is no longer possible in the church setting.

While attending a training program would be optimal, videos of a training workshop that I led are available online.[6] I would recommend watching those and reading the materials available at the program website. I would also recommend that this program be delivered by teams of two or three people. There are kits of all the stories but Easter available for sale that contain all the underlays and wooden pieces needed for each service. Scripts for each service are also contained in the kit. Scripts and patterns for figures are also on the website mentioned above.[7]

In the ideal world this worship would be done weekly and the stories rotated by the liturgical season. The Advent/Christmas story would be told during Advent and Christmas season. In ordinary times, the story of the Good Shepherd and Jesus and Zacchaeus is used with the green

---

6 www.spiritualityandaging.org/sensing-the-sacred

7 For information about instituting this program in your setting, contact me at: sensingthesacred@gmail.com.

underlay. During Lent, the story of Jesus and Zacchaeus is used with a purple underlay. The Easter story is told during Eastertide.

This program is not the easiest to use. It requires thought and preparation and memorization. But, I have found that in using it you come into a spiritual communion with those you are worshiping with. I think it is one good way to provide volunteers with a deeply meaningful experience, and an experience that lessons the fears and stigma that so many have connected with Alzheimer's disease. In using it in memory care units, I have often found that when I started and greeted every one by name the group was not centered and some were much more there than others. But by the end of the service, when I went around and gave each an individual blessing, they were much more present than they had been at the beginning and often blessed me in response. Staff confirmed that the peacefulness of the service stayed with them for several hours.

References

Hanson, R., Mabry, J., and Williams, R. (2003) 'Companioning people with dementia.' *Journal of Spiritual Direction* 9, 3, 45–54.

Keane, B. and Ustick, K. (2003) 'Montessori principles work for Alzheimer's, based on an interview with Bill Keane and Kathleen Ustick.' *Nursing Homes Magazine*. Retrieved from www.iadvanceseniorcare.com/article/montessori-principles-work-alzheimers on October 10, 2018.

McFadden, S., Ingram, M., and Olson Baldauf, C. (2010) 'Actions, feelings, and values: Foundations of meaning and personhood in dementia.' *Journal of Religious Gerontology* 11, 3–4, 67–86.

Stewart, S. and Berryman, J.W. (1989) *Young Children and Worship*. Louisville, KY: Westminster John Knox Press.

A Layperson's Guide to Improvised Worship

Finding Spiritual Expression through Intentional Connections

Elizabeth R. Reinert, MED (Interdenominational Christian)

One of the most effective ways to build a bridge with someone with advanced dementia who is living in a care facility is by visiting regularly. Even if you are not clergy, a person of faith can encourage spiritual interactions when alone with one person or in a group. You may be there as a family member, friend, or volunteer. When verbal communication fails, sitting with the person can speak volumes. Spending unhurried time and attention shows the person with dementia that you value him or her. This is sometimes referred to as "the ministry of presence."

Careful observation on your part may be required to detect some way to further "warm up" to the person before trying to offer any spiritual connection or attempt a more meaningful encounter. This may be achieved by utilizing the "love language" of the person you are trying to connect with.

Dr. Gary Chapman, coauthor of *Keeping Love Alive as Memories Fade* (2016), has determined that everyone has one or more "love languages." They are 1) physical touch, 2) quality time, 3) words of affirmation, 4) receiving gifts, and 5) acts of service. Keeping these in mind, holding the person's hand may help promote a connection, coupled by focusing on the person and not hurrying any agenda you may have. Knowing the person's history helps one think of positive things to say about his or her life story, interests, or accomplishments. A small token of food, flowers, a soft stuffed animal, etc. may be readily received. Or the person may appreciate some assistance such as picking up a slipper that has fallen onto the floor and returning it to an exposed foot. Using all five languages has a better chance of hitting the mark than just guessing and trying one or two—with potentially striking results. Helping a person feel loved may open doors for deeper engagement. I frequently used hand holding and singing to get my mother's attention when I was her caregiver. She always welcomed food, special gifts, or just hearing of her life and family, which helped her become more aware of my presence, especially if we were alone together, away from the public gatherings and noise.

Awareness of how you are feeling when you visit is important. Are you relaxed, cheerful, and attentive? Or are you feeling somewhat sad, distracted, or uncertain of how to proceed? Often your comfort level or mood will be reflected back to you, setting the tone of your time together. Consider when a visit to a long-term care facility is most welcome. Whether you are visiting an assisted living, memory care, or skilled care facility, the lengthy period between lunch and supper is usually a good time to visit. The more frequent your visits are to a long-term care facility, the more willing the residents are to engage with you.

In my experience as a caregiver to my mother, moving her over time to all levels of care, I had the advantage of being with her and her fellow residents on an almost daily basis. Even though I had no prior relationship with her "neighbors," because we were together at mealtime, in activities, or just sitting together in common areas, we became familiar and comfortable with one another. Familiarity breeds opportunity for all kinds of interaction, including improvised worship. Being aware of the simple needs of the residents takes observation, followed by action. This is helpful to the residents and the staff who over time may forget you are a visitor, helping you to blend in with everyone else.

This proved true with many of my new friends who had dementia. I grew to know which rooms folks belonged in and what their daily habits were. In the memory care facility, all residents would be seated or walking in the common space, where there were recliners for relaxing in addition to tables and chairs for mealtime and other activities. The long afternoons between lunch and dinner relied on napping with the sound of the TV to pass the time. Residents would become restless and perhaps begin to wander into trouble, trying to find the way out or mistake a neighbor's room or bathroom for their own.

So I would invite anyone available to join my mother, my aunt, and me at a round dinner table for some social interaction. This was not scheduled on an activity calendar, and I had no agenda other than to help pass the time in a positive way, creating an atmosphere of happiness and camaraderie.

Rolling a medium-sized rubber ball back and forth between our group kept us focused and occupied. Singing all kinds of songs together kept the interaction upbeat, evoking laughter and playfulness. Having a folder on hand full of the words to songs, poems, and word games helped everyone participate. We might begin with popular songs from earlier eras and move onto familiar hymns. This might lead to offering a familiar Bible verse or prayer and even reminiscing about spiritual experiences, church involvement, and beliefs.

All this interaction created trust and love between us. People with dementia may not remember what you said, but they will remember how you made them feel. I found that it was better to just go with the flow, paying attention to body language and mood, while gently leading with purpose. Where did I want to lead them? To a place of contentment and safety, to a place that draws on their history, to an awareness of respect for their lives, and to a feeling of connection with God and others.

Gaining another's trust over time allows for very special interactions. The first time this happened to me, I acted on a prompting in my spirit. I had passed a lady's room on my way out to the car, knowing that the resident inside, with whom I had developed a close relationship, was said to be dying. As I sat in my car, I realized that I might never see this person alive again. I considered both her and her daughter my friends. A song began to form in my mind and I began to sing it out loud. I decided to go back in and see my friend one last time.

I entered her room, passing the daughter, who was standing in the hallway talking on the phone. This was a rather bold move, but I was compelled to accomplish my mission. There she lay, eyes closed, fan set up at the foot of the bed, blowing cool air to help her breathe. I laid my hand on her hands that were clasped on her chest under the blanket and began to sing the song that had come to mind while I was in my car. As I sang, the daughter joined me by the bedside and we both gazed upon her dying mother's face.

To our surprise, her mother began to move her lips and silently mouth the words—all of them. So I started another praise and worship song, which she also knew. The daughter asked, "How did you know to sing these songs? Momma sang in the choir and knows these by heart." This moment gave us both such a precious connection with her mother, with each other, and with God that I determined in the future to continue to move where the Spirit led.

Her mother never opened her eyes again and died the next day. The daughter never forgot the experience and eventually joined my church and gave her life to Christ. Our shared experience of improvised worship occurred only as a result of being sensitive to the present situation and acting on it.

If I noticed a minister come visit a resident who was in bed with eyes closed, under hospice care, entering the final stage of life, I might accompany him to the bedside. One particular time, sensing the minister wasn't sure what to do, I began singing "Jesus Loves Me." Standing on the other side of the bed, he joined me in song. The woman we were singing to lifted her eyebrows in response to the sound of our voices. Knowing she was listening, he then said a prayer and left satisfied that his visit had been worthwhile.

Allowing the mood in the room to dictate your approach is critical. Perhaps the television has been spewing terrible news all morning and the residents have absorbed it as their own bad news. Upon hearing the news of the Sandy Hook shootings that replayed all afternoon for everyone to hear, I remember one lady worried and fretted about her children the rest of the day.

It's not unusual to have staff shortages at care facilities, causing delays in the usual schedule, creating cross tempers and restless residents. On the other hand, the mood might be happy, with the sun shining in the windows and pleasant music playing in the background. The following story is how a particular afternoon played out without any preconceived notions. We were just being together, as we often were, in a day room, passing the time when an opportunity for improvised worship occurred.

It all started with "Rudolph the Red-Nosed Reindeer."

The commercial on the television advertised the favorite Christmas movie in the background noise of the nursing home day room. I looked across from where I was sitting and made eye contact with a beautiful lady who sat in a wheelchair and was looking at me with her clear eyes. "Rudolph the red-nosed reindeer..." I declared. Together we continued in unison: "...had a very shiny nose, and if you ever saw it, you would even say it glowed."

Not wanting to lose the momentum, I started singing "Frosty the Snowman." My fellow singer joined me again, and we sang all the words we could remember. She knew more of them than I did. Smiling and laughing at our achievement, I searched for another familiar song. "Deck the halls with boughs of holly," I began, and we finished together. Searching again, I started, "We wish you a merry Christmas," and again she joined me, without hesitation. It was almost as if she had been waiting for this opportunity. Her countenance was eager and engaged.

A young man by the door kept silent but expressed his joy in the unexpected eruption by occasionally turning to look at us with a big smile. By now, I was starting to run out of Christmas selections. After "Silent Night" and "Away in a Manger," silence fell in the room. My pretty friend said, "For God so loved the world that He gave his only begotten Son so that whoever believes in Him will have everlasting life, John 3.16." Taking her cue, I began to sing, "Jesus loves me, this I know."

Jo, another resident, joined in while looking out the window as if she could see another place and time. She walked over to the couch and sat down and said, "Now we are starting to have church. Yes, Lord, Jesus loves me. You know that's the truth." Jo was beginning to tell what she believed. I initiated the Lord's Prayer. Jo took it and continued, so I stopped speaking while she completed the prayer.

"That's right," said my clear-eyed friend.

"Yes," I agreed, "Jesus loves us, thank you, Jesus."

We were sharing a moment that transcended our location and situation. Above the occasional clatter from the hallway that made my wheelchair-bound friend wince, our spirits rose to another place.

We held on to it with our collective experience from days gone past, yet we were present, all at the same time. We each shared what we carried inside us and found beauty together. The feeling of love permeated the room.

This type of scenario would repeat itself many times in many different ways over the years caring for my loved ones. Allowing for time, friendship, and awareness, one can introduce spiritual experiences in the most unexpected moments. Seizing the opportunity often produced the most memorable moments for me and left a pleasant mood for all involved.

A dear lady who lived in the room next to my mom noticed my routine of leaving at a certain time in the afternoon. She began to park her wheelchair in the hallway by her door so that I would pass her on my way out. As a result, we developed a friendship that would last after both my mother and aunt died. Over time, we learned about each other's life histories, daily activities, and our faith, which turned to sharing favorite Bible verses.

As her health deteriorated and my friend began to forget who I was, I would still arrive armed with a bag of activities to introduce during our visit. She enjoyed hearing me sing songs to her but would not join in.

When I would read the 23rd Psalm, however, she would join me as the words came to her mind. We would read it again and, by the third time, she would be reciting from memory the entire verse by herself. She was always very pleased by that and believed I was visiting from her church to brighten her day. Although I was a layperson and a recent friend, I was able to offer spiritual food that fed both our spirits.

Helping someone or a group of people who live with memory loss enjoy meaningful spiritual practices takes leadership, sensitivity, and love. The times with my mother and new friends in memory care gathered around the table, singing songs, and rolling the ball to each other, and in long-term care passing the time in the day room together, allowed for opportunities to share our faith in expressive ways. In every stage of the disease process, people with dementia can enjoy friendship, give and receive love, and maintain emotional connections. Both you and the participants can find the holiest of moments through Spirit-led improvised worship.

Reference

Barr, D., Shaw, E.G., and Chapman, G. (2016) *Keeping Love Alive as Memories Fade: The Five Love Languages and the Alzheimer's Journey.* Chicago, IL: Northfield Publishing.

Familiar Hymns, Prayers, and Scriptures to Use in a Small Group Setting for Memory-Impaired Adults

Elizabeth R. Reinert, MEd (Interdenominational Christian)

Meeting with a small group of residents in a memory care facility using the following songs, scriptures, and the Lord's Prayer allows for deep memories to surface and be shared. Whether you want to lead an organized church service or just want to add to your repertoire of activities to pull out at any time, the following is tried and true.

You can easily find the words to the songs online or in a hymnal. You may want to have several large print copies of the songs available for those who can follow along.

Begin with John 3.16, a familiar scripture, and move through the list. Any changes or additions the participants may offer are welcomed and don't need to be corrected. Take your time and observe each response, allowing for contributions to be given and heard.

Keep in mind that the attention span of your participants may require adjustments in your choices. You may need to shorten or alter the flow to keep everyone's interest. What works well one day may not the next. Remain flexible and keep the focus on the folks you are ministering to rather than accomplishing your plan.

Your time could go something like this:

1. Read "For God so loved the world, that he gave his only Son, that whoever believes in him should not perish but have eternal life" (John 3.16, *English Standard Version*).

2. Sing "Blessed Assurance," "Jesus Loves Me," and "Nothing But the Blood."

3. Read "Do not let your heart be troubled; believe in God, believe also in Me. In My Father's house are many dwelling places; if it were not so, I would have told you; for I go to prepare a place for

you. If I go and prepare a place for you, I will come again and receive you to Myself, that where I am, there you may be also" (John 14.1–3, *New American Standard Bible*).

You may want to talk about what this personally means to you, inviting other comments. Perhaps you may just thank the Lord for his comforting promises, leading the way to talk about His grace and the next song choice.

4. Sing "Amazing Grace."
5. Recite "The Lord's Prayer."
6. Sing "How Great Thou Art" and "In the Garden."
7. Read "Trust in the Lord with all your heart and do not lean on your own understanding. In all your ways acknowledge Him, and He will make your paths straight" (Proverbs 3.5–6, *New American Standard Bible*).
8. Sing "I'll Fly Away" and "The Doxology."

Especially for Easter

Sing "He Lives," "The Old Rugged Cross," and "Because He Lives."

Especially for Christmas

Sing "Away in a Manger," "Hark the Herald Angels Sing," and "Joy to the World." With so many Christmas songs to choose from, participants may offer some of their own preferences. To add some fun, include favorites like "Rudolph the Red-Nosed Reindeer," "Deck the Halls," and "Jingle Bells," and end with "We Wish You a Merry Christmas."

Use all or parts of these songs and scriptures in an intentional, organized service and also as an improvised worship experience when the moment is right. Participants most often join in, singing the songs and reciting the familiar verses. If you see someone reciting a passage from memory, try initiating the verse again, then allow him or her to take the lead. If another song arises from someone in the group, join in as well. You may finish the service with something particularly meaningful to your group or locale. One southern tradition we have is saying, "God is good," and the response is "All the time." And then we say, "All the time," and the response is "God is good."

Tapping these spiritual memories allows for meaningful moments both personally and interactively. A sense of belonging and communion can arise within the group, renewing and uplifting the spirit of all involved.

Thank You, Lord, For My Right Mind

Dr. Pernessa C. Seele (Christian)

It is Sunday morning. It is the only day of the week that you can spend at least two hours with my mother when she is "in her right mind." I grew up listening to the "old folks" praying and thanking God for allowing them to "wake up this morning in my right mind." Of course at this point on my life's journey, I am now very aware of why the supplication of their prayers was so sincere and intense.

My mother has Alzheimer's. She is filled with laughter and joy even in the midst of this dreadful disease. She often jokes that she does not have Alzheimer's but part-timer's. Such might be true if you ever attend Sunday morning worship with her. From the rising of the sun on Sunday morning through the process of getting dressed, getting in the car, and answering her questions a thousand and one times, she is lost in her memory of what is happening around her within seconds. But she is happy and eager each time you answer her inquiring thought, "Where are we going?" There are no words to express her joy when she receives the answer over and over again, "We are going to church!"

Experiencing her happiness when she walks through the church doors into the world that she knows and is 100 percent present and comfortable in is a miracle for everyone around her to experience. It is the rhythm of the African American Church cadence, the foundation of her faith, and the omnipotent, omnipresence, and omniscient elements of God that delivers my mom's memory back to her when she enters the church sanctuary. She sings every song with her thundering vocals just as she did when she was the lead singer in the local gospel group over 40 years ago singing The Caravan's "We'll Go Sweeping Through the City." Hands clappin' and foot stompin', my mom leans back and stretches her sight toward heaven when the choir sings Walker Hawkins' "Going Up Yonder" or the soulful gospel lyrics of "Take My Hand, Precious Lord," as written and recorded by Rev. Thomas A. Dorsey. In church, she is home. The rituals of worship are so familiar to her. With no support, she follows the instructions to turn in your Bible to any and every book, chapter, and verse. She knows every word to old hymns and those ancient songs of the Black Church that too often did not make it to a page in a book, such as:

Sweet Home, Sweet Home, Sweet Home, My Lord!
Lord, I wonder, if I'll ever get Home!

From the moment of the Call to Worship to the Benediction, she is in her right mind and present with all her surroundings. However, once she departs from the sanctuary, crossing the door steps of the church, she is back in a world of memory loss and no recall of where she has been for the past two hours or the joy that we all witnessed flowing from her.

The African American Church—its embracing congregants and thundering pulpit—is so important in this era of our living when the rates of Alzheimer's disease among African American men and women are among the highest in our nation. For only two hours per week, my mother's soul, which has no memory loss, re-connects with her mind through the familiar rhythms of the Black Church experience. Her communion, as she partakes of the bread and wine, gives a gloried shout to her testimony about the blood of Jesus, which brings tears to her eyes. The response of our church must be one of commitment to our elderly and all those living with Alzheimer's. As our Christian education and youth departments have flourished for centuries, the Black Church must now create structures that support and embrace our elderly. Our congregations must find creative ways to address the needs of those living with Alzheimer's and other chronic diseases as well as create and support a system of healthy aging throughout our life span. Caregiving, a staple of the Black experience, must now be re-ignited with special attention and resources for those individuals who are in the trenches of caring for those unable to care for themselves. Equally important: African American faith leaders must work to re-connect our institutions as caring stations of all persons—young and old.

Note: Memory Sunday is always the second Sunday in June. Established by The Balm In Gilead, Memory Sunday provides resources, such as *The Book of Alzheimer's for African American Congregations*, to support caregivers and persons living with Alzheimer's throughout the entire year.

For over 30 years, The Balm In Gilead has worked to prevent diseases and improve the health of individuals by providing support to faith and other institutions in areas of program design, implementation, and evaluation, all of which strengthen their capacity to deliver programs and services that contribute to the elimination of health disparities. For more information: www.balmingilead.org.

Spiritual Metamorphosis

Tryn Rose Seley (Christian, New Church)

> Crying may last for a night. But joy comes in the morning. (Psalm 30.5; *International Children's Bible*)

I love seeing people re-emerge from behind the covers and constraints our earthly bodies might encounter. I've led worship services for all ages and abilities, and currently lead "Mindful Art" at an adult day program, where the participants re-emerge all the time when we sing, tell life stories, worship, and create art together.

My brother Martin had grand mal seizures every other day of his nine years of life on this earth, and petit mal seizures the rest of the time, starting at about 18 months. He persisted amongst these constant lightning strikes, though many things were affected. I was a year older. His tender soul emerged as he'd greet us with "Hi...hi...hi..." in his gentle voice or share his love of butterflies, calling them "bu-thu-thy" for butterfly. Lately, I've been enjoying monarch and queen caterpillars on the native milkweed plants here in Arizona and he comes to mind often.

I learned from Martin that he was "in there" beyond the layers of difficulty, and his presence in my life was extremely formative. I have pursued careers that recognize a person is "in there," and operate from that belief; I've enjoyed seeing people emerge from their cocoons, so to speak, when regarded with compassion, love, and respect. From leading music for church camps in the Laurel Mountain Ridge of the Appalachians for children with special needs to creating programs for elders with dementia in the Rockies and in the Delaware Water Gap, I've had the joy of seeing people burst forth from their cocoons to become the beautiful butterflies they are meant to be, even if only for a moment. That moment is precious and important. I believe they will become fully themselves again after passing into the spiritual world, free from the earthly constraints, so I try to remember this as I interact with these blessed souls.

As a music therapist and professional photographer, I understand the power of using one photo, one song, one story to connect with another and open the door for a shared and meaningful experience of Divine worship. It's a blessing to see someone who feels troubled, anxious, or frustrated sail through their challenging emotions and feel relieved, relaxed, and connected. It happens over and over again when you *start the conversation and see what emerges.* If you know one thing about the person you're serving—"You were some lawyer in your day" or "You made quilts for your children and grandchildren" or "You are a master gardener" or "You sang in your church choir"—then you open the door to a person's memories, and they may come spilling out in a beautiful way!

I found that such simple statements can bring back feelings of pride and delight in one's lifetime of accomplishments and allow us to transition to a place of one-to-one worship. This can happen when you strive to build authentic relationships, seeing those whom you serve as people first, and valuing them for who they truly are. Not everyone will be able to engage in and benefit from large group worship experiences, but you may make amazing connections with folks individually that can help them connect with their faith.

One effective way of doing this is by telling people some of their own life story. For example, a friend of mine who had been a church organist was well into dementia in her older years. She had inspired me as a young adult. At women's retreats, she consulted her self-made card catalog containing her favorite quotes from the Bible, which set me on a life-long path of collecting quotes and inviting participants to share their favorite quotes in many worship contexts. She had forgotten she had done this, forgotten she had taught yoga and played hymns for hundreds of people over the years. The key: her daughter had created a montage including photos of her at the organ of all six congregations; she started the conversation. When I visited her, I would say, "You played the organ for so many years. You inspired a lot of people. Thank you." She'd say "I did?…I did that?" and I'd show her the pictures, name the congregations in Ohio, Arizona, Pennsylvania… and she'd marvel at the story of her life! She smiled, felt comforted, felt remembered and valued. Later, even as the dementia progressed, if she was invited to sit at a keyboard, she could play these hymns again; her muscle memory kicked in and she radiated angelic beauty once more! Her true self emerged again in those moments! Years later, my sister and I visited her in the midnight hour because the family let us know she was distressed and unhappy. When we shared how she inspired us both on our life paths, sang her favorite song ("Seek Ye First the Kingdom of God… Allelu, Allelujah…"), and gave her a hands-on blessing, the light and love of God shone out of her eyes, she sang along, and looked restored and peaceful as she settled down and went to sleep.

Another woman I had met just one time before, when she was laughing and playing adapted basketball with a group, was in anguish and pain the next time, lying on the couch at the adult day program. I played sacred music and created worship for a group of 25, then came to her side, held her hand, listened, and said, "I'm so sorry you're feeling sad and lonely. I love you. The Lord is with you always. God will not leave you comfortless." She was not as outwardly comforted as I hoped, but I could see that she did rest a little easier before I left that day. She passed away soon after, which seemed like the ultimate "rest" and effect one could wish for. She stayed in her cocoon when I was with her, but was released from it with a little love and attention to help send her on her journey. I did not know it would be her last day; it was a blessing to spend it with her, listening to her, loving her, and sharing God's love with her.

You never know what will be your last day, or anyone else's last day, or what spiritual need might be there for you to minister to. If you take a moment to see the longing for human and Divine connection in the eyes of those you serve, and just stay, be present, listen, and tell them you love them and God loves them, that can make all the difference for you and the one you care for. Know that your work is worthwhile, and that God is with you in your daily efforts.

My caregiver book, phone app, and music, storytelling, and art-creating sessions are all based on this idea of *starting the conversation* and improvising with what emerges. Don't ask a question; make a statement: "I remember my first music director; she invited me to lead 'Jesus Loves Me.' I've been leading music ever since," or "I loved lighting candles at Christmas Eve service with my family." It gives the listener a place to start with their own stories of church or worship or other spiritual experiences as well as current spiritual needs. When a person seems absent, you may be surprised when a stream of memories bubbles back to the surface when you start the story.

Here are some other possible starting points. The Serenity Prayer is well known and loved. The rosary is well established and practiced. Meditations, yoga practices, qigong, and Tai Chi are long-standing practices. Any of these systems can re-anchor someone who is flailing in anxiety and sadness and spiritual neediness. Every person from every faith background I've ever met knows "Amazing Grace," "Swing Low, Sweet Chariot," and "Joy to the World." So, I sing them every session, and the smiles shine like the sun rising in the East.

Structure for a one-to-one visit

Greet someone in an open-ended way: "Hello, I'm (name). I'm glad to see you today." He or she will respond with happiness, sadness, or maybe grumpiness. Then you'll know where you are starting. You may just listen and then respond. "I'm here to be with you." "I'm glad" or "I'm sorry" or "I love you and God loves you" are all good responses.

I bring a folder of resources to utilize and share. These can be helpful for interacting with a person:

- Bible passage index cards. I can:
  - read one aloud
  - offer him or her one to draw, read, consider, discuss
  - ask for a favorite Bible quote or prayer in case he or she can share it
  - read familiar scriptures and omit a word, letting him or her fill it in: "The Lord is my...(wait for it) ... Shepherd!"
- Cards with a simple love note format to leave in the room in case he or she is asleep or unable to connect on that day: for example, "God loves you and so do I" or "May the Lord bless you and keep you" or "God is a Sun and a Shield...God is with you always." A person can see this later, gain some comfort, or feel the surprise of a gift, and you can read it again the next time you visit. Family, friends, and other visitors can also enjoy such a token of love and share it with the person. Helpful hint: make two identical cards and bring yours back for a follow-up visit, in case the one you delivered goes missing.
- Life story prompts from a game, or from various resources: "What's your favorite place: mountains, ocean, rivers, grasslands?" Start the conversation—"I love the ocean, picking up shells, and hearing the sea birds; my heart is in Florida"—and see what emerges from their memories.
- The Sheet Game: literally, a sheet (easy to fold up and carry) with written topics of conversation, and a beanbag to decide which one to discuss: First car, First church, School days, Pets, Awards, Projects, etc.

A group format that can be as easy as "A, B, C"

A: Welcome the group, open a Bible or other sacred text, and sing! Best choices I've chosen that most people know are "Amazing Grace," "Swing Low, Sweet Chariot," and "Joy to the World."

B: Be flexible, offer variety. As with one-to-one resources:

- read scriptural quotes aloud
- read and let participants finish the quote: "The Lord is my... *Shepherd!*"
- let discussion ensue: "When I think of the Lord as my Shepherd, I feel safe and secure, protected, loved. What does the Shepherd image mean to you?"

Also, for this section of the service, you can invite family members, children, local church choirs, or surprise visitors who may be present to contribute a sacred song, a reading, a performance. People living with dementia may like to play a hymn if a piano or guitar is available, or lead a Bible reading and prayer, especially if you offer this opportunity to participate and contribute.

C: Close the gathering with a song, and bless all participants with "May the Lord bless you and keep you" or "Peace be with you." A familiar tradition is the passing of the peace: invite the group to say goodbye with shaking of hands and exchanging "Peace be with you" and "Also with you."

When I worked for care communities, I created an Evening Vespers service. Many are restless in the evening, not settled down for the night yet. We'd gather and sing "Amazing Grace," "You Are My Sunshine," "Down in the Valley," "Red River Valley," "All Through the Night," "Silent Night," and more... It meant that people could calm down into the evening hours, feeling more at peace with God and themselves. Caregivers could also assist one person at a time to bed, a blessing for them too. The transformation from busy day to quiet night was wonderful to see.

So, may you always recognize a person is still "in there" beyond the layers of difficulty, and create sacred spaces of shared worship that spiritually nurture everyone who enters. If you stay present, observe carefully, and respond to someone with compassion, love, and respect, you may see that butterfly emerge from its cocoon and catch a glimpse of that angel in the making.

Making God "Real"

Using the Senses to "Experience" Scripture

Dr. Jane Marie Thibault (Roman Catholic/United Methodist)

Making God's message in Scripture relevant to the lives of adults suffering from dementia can be a real challenge and requires a degree of creativity. If you have ever designed a child's Sunday school class, think about how you used all of the senses and body movements to get the story across, to make it real and very concrete for the children. Getting the message across didn't rely on hearing alone, as it is for "grown-ups" attending a traditional service—it was a whole body experience!

Older adults who have participated in a faith community at some time in their lives, especially those who have been members of faith formation classes as children, are most likely to remember the frequently told and the most dramatic stories from the Hebrew and Christian Scriptures. These stories are embedded in their early memories and may be able to be accessed for spiritual care, especially if they can be related to their current life. For example, Genesis 12, wherein 75-year-old Abraham is instructed to leave his secure home and abundant lands to travel into the unknown, can be related to the need to leave one's beloved home to live institutionally. Genesis 17.15–22 and Genesis 18.1–15, the stories of God's promise to Abraham and Sarah that they will finally have a son at ages 90 and 100, are dramatic and even funny and can also be used to point out how God delivers on his promises—even when all hope seems lost.

The spiritual practice of encountering God in Scripture has its origin in Ignatian/Jesuit theology, where the reader or hearer is invited to enter the story as one of the "characters." This method of prayer was first taught by St. Ignatius of Loyola in the 16th century, who called the practice "composition of place." It is also called the "prayer of active imagination." It is very similar to an actor taking on the role of a character in a play. The purpose of its use as a prayer method is to break down the barriers between God and the person who prays, to allow the person to enter into the lives of Biblical characters and those whose lives they touched. Many of the stories in the Hebrew and the Christian Scriptures lend themselves to this type of prayer method, which can be engaged in as an individual, one-on-one with a person, or in small groups. For example, if you are a pastor presiding at a Christmas service in a nursing home for a small group of people with dementia, or if you are a caregiver on Christmas Eve, you might do something like this:

- Play the music of one of the best-known hymns, e.g. "Silent Night."
- Invite attendees to sing along—first stanza only—two or three times.
- Choose Luke's narrative of the birth of Jesus and re-write it to simplify the story—or read the story from a child's Bible. Read it slowly.
- Ask the group the following questions (there are many more that can be asked) and wait for answers:
  - What do you think it was like in Bethlehem that night?
  - Was it cold, crowded, smelly?
  - Did you ever wonder what it was like being a member of the crowd or being Mary, Joseph, or the inn-keeper?
- Now tell the group you are going to read the passage again. Ask each person to imagine themselves as a member of the crowd in Bethlehem that night, and re-read the passage. When you have finished it, ask each person as they imagine themselves as a member of the Bethlehem crowd:
  - Are you a man or woman?
  - Are you a grown-up or a child?
  - What do you *see* all around you?
  - What do you *hear* all around you?
  - What do you *smell*?
  - What do you *feel*?
  - What do you *taste*?
- Go around the room, giving each person a chance to say what their experience of being a member of the crowd in Bethlehem was like.

- The above exercise may be long enough, with enough content, depending on whether people are able to respond. If no one responds, tell them how *you* experienced being a part of the crowd, sharing your answers to all of the above questions.

If there is more time and the people aren't needing to leave, proceed with the rest of the story.

- Ask each person to imagine themselves as Mary, using all their senses. What was she wearing? Was she warm or cold? What did the air smell like? Was it night time or still light? Was she just starting her labor pains or were they coming fast? Did she hurt? What was she feeling—was she frightened? Excited? Was she annoyed with Joseph because he hadn't made reservations for a room? Was she exhausted?
- When all Joseph could find for Mary's protection was a cave full of animals being sheltered for the night, what do you think Mary was thinking? Feeling? Did she wish her mother was there? Do you think she wished she had never agreed to be the mother of Jesus? How would *you* have felt if this had happened to you when you were 14? What was your life like when you were 14?
- If the room is full of men, have them take the character of Joseph and ask similar questions.

If they won't or can't respond, share your own experience of being Mary or Joseph.

This exercise of "living" Scripture can be done:

- individually—caregiver or person in earlier stages of dementia by him/herself
- as a dyad—pastor, lay volunteer, or caregiver with person with dementia
- in a group setting (as shown above).

There is no "right" or "wrong" way to practice "living" Scripture. In whatever way you can, use the senses to help activate the person's spiritual imagination. The purpose is to create or sustain an emotional bond with God by entering into the stories.

Chapter 3

MINISTERING TO SPECIFIC FAITH COMMUNITIES

The Sacred Circle of Life

Native Americans and Dementia

Rev. Cynthia J. Abrams (October 11, 1960–January 11, 2019) (United Methodist)

Native Americans number 4.5 million according to the last U.S. Census. There are 573 federally recognized tribes as well as many state-recognized tribes. Native American/American Indian people live on reservations and tribal allotment lands, and in cities, suburbs, and rural areas, across this nation. The largest populations of Native Americans are in Oklahoma and California, but there are many other states that have significant populations as well. It is estimated that just 2 percent of Native Americans are Christian. The vast majority of Native people practice their traditional tribal religious ways. It's important to keep in mind that Native Americans are not monolithic. There is great diversity between individual tribes, even those that are related to each other, such as the six tribes of the Iroquois confederacy. Each tribe has distinct traditional rituals and religious ceremonies, and even Christian Natives may have distinct worship traditions from one place to another. Many of the traditional rituals and ceremonies are private and not accessible to non-Natives. There are a few ceremonies that are public, usually related to public gatherings of Native people, such as the Iroquois social dances, pow wows, some Apache Crown dances, etc.

Alzheimer's disease and dementia are not common topics among Native people.[1] This is primarily due to cultural mores and the extended intergenerational familial system common amongst tribes. The extended family plays a critical role in the structure of tribal society. The extended family is equally important to the nuclear family, and in some cases roles are more important outside the nuclear family, particularly if the nuclear family is experiencing instability for some reason. Commonplace among the extended family is taking care of the

1 *Editors' note*: Mayeda *et al.* (2016) cite a research summary comparing dementia incidence across six racial and ethnic groups. Native Americans had an incidence of 22.2 cases per 1000 people, compared with 26.6 for African Americans and 19.3 for white Americans. Thus, Native Americans are at an increased risk for dementia.

Elders, since a key value among Native people is that Elders have revered status. They are given a primary role in the teaching of oral tradition, in solving family problems, in providing guidance, and in the upbringing of children. However, if the Elder is ill, the extended family steps in and quickly develops a process to care for and protect the Elder. There is much privacy in the midst of these situations. Other Native people respect the privacy but provide a level of communication that ensures others in the tribe are praying for or providing rituals to cover the Elder's illness.

One of the challenges with this approach is that early intervention for Alzheimer's may suffer. Outside resources may not be trusted due to the long history of mistrust of people "outside" the tribal membership and an element of mistrust for Western medicine. There are exceptions to this, such as the Indian Health Service (IHS) on reservations, including non-Indian doctors, nurses, and medical personnel who service the IHS clinics on reservations and Indian lands. Another resource may be trusted non-Indian and Native clergy who serve in a predominantly Indian area. Each of these resources is greatly dependent on in-depth cultural training sensitive to Native people and to the particular tribe they serve.

Most Native people think of life in a circular and contiguous fashion. Everything is connected and everyone is a relation. The Lakota Sioux call this Mitakuye Oyasin, defined as "all my relations," meaning we are all related and we are all interconnected. To me, as a Christian who is Native, Paul's first letter to the church in Corinth aptly illustrates a similar understanding: "For just as the body is one and has many members, and all the members of the body, though many, are one body, so it is with Christ" (1 Corinthians 12.12, *New Revised Standard Version*). One way of conceptualizing this is through the Sacred Circle of Life. There is no beginning and no end to the circle. Each direction on the circle, North, South, East, and West, contributes to a rhythmic way of life where everything is connected and in harmony. The Sacred Circle of Life teaches us that we all share an equal place in the circle. Thus, in cases of Elders with dementia, they are a part of the circle too, ever giving, ever receiving, despite cognitive/communicative limitations. Even non-communicative Elders are important to the connection in community and may be present at communal events. The Creator/God is found at the center of the Sacred Circle. We hear God's voice in the winds, in the Four Directions. Through the center of the circle passes the Four Directions dividing the circle into four separate, but equal, parts representing a distinct phase of the life cycle.

The Sacred Circle of Life has neither beginning nor end. The circle reflects our relationship to the infinite Creation and Creator; thus, the Circle of Life represents the unity of all things.

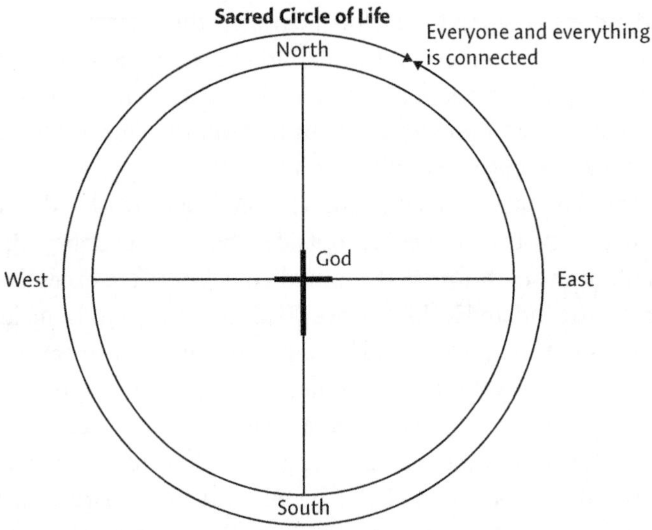

Cultural training for clergy and other church leadership is essential in ministering with Native people and broaching sensitive subjects such as Alzheimer's disease or dementia. Here are some key learnings from my experience.

Native people value:

- *Cooperation*—Working together. This includes tribal initiatives and extended family priorities; both are important to the overall health of the tribal community.
- *Harmony*—Working to find the centering and spiritual side to situations. Being in conflict is not valued. The challenge is that if people disagree over health concerns it can be difficult to come to resolution.
- *Modesty*—Physical and emotional modesty is important. For example, it is important not to tout your achievements. Another example of this is that one must wear appropriate clothing/jewelry that does not draw attention to oneself.

- *Religion* is in every part of life: in the phases of life, in health and disease, from birth to death, as portrayed in the Sacred Circle of Life above.
- *Silence/Listening*—There is power in silence! There will often be long periods of silence in a conversation with a Native person. It's important not to fill those silences. This is where discussion with a Native family about an Elder with Alzheimer's disease or dementia can be tripped up. For Western society, silence can be interpreted as acquiescence. To ensure accurate expectations and understandings occur, it is critically important to listen and be silent.
- *Control is given to the Creator*—There is the key value that life has a natural rhythm to it. Therefore, Native American caregivers do not expect to control the process of caring for an Elder.
- *Revered Elders* in the tribe have a place in decision-making processes even if they are not biologically related. Traditional healers, Elders with special standing, contribute invaluable and culturally appropriate interventions. Even if the person is Christian, the traditional rituals are usually important to the family and individual. Also, when an Elder is speaking, everyone must listen and not interrupt.
- *Language*—In some cases the primary language in the home may be a tribal language. There is a deep sense of connection with the tribal language. However, in urban settings most Native people speak English as well. On reservations, people may speak English and their tribal language interchangeably. On more remote reservations, there is a likelihood that the tribal language is the primary language.

Songs and prayers

Tribal hymns are important touchstones for families. They are sung at special gatherings and for different phases of life, from birth to death. Getting in touch with a local Native clergyperson or traditional Elder to invite Native singers, drummers, flute players, etc. can be important moments for the person with Alzheimer's disease or dementia. They may remember their tribal language or begin to sing tribal songs at the most surprising moments. I have witnessed a non-verbal person suddenly begin speaking their language and singing on their deathbed.

Prayers

Embrace and Celebrate the Sacred Circle of Life

We celebrate the contributions Native People of this land have made to God's Church. We learn from them that life is a sacred circle, of which there is no beginning and no end. We are all a part of that circle, ever contributing, ever receiving. Native Americans teach us that as a part of the circle we must care for all of God's creation. We know that God's creation includes all that is a part of this earth, the wingeds, the two-leggeds, plants and the sky. We remember and worship God the Creator throughout our daily lives, even as we look at a tree, the grass or the sky. For Genesis reminds us that God looked at everything and was very pleased. We embrace and celebrate the Sacred Circle of Life.

Cynthia Abrams (1989; a prayer I wrote and published in *Voices: Native American Hymns and Other Worship Resources* (Hofstra 1992))

We Are All Related

We share our stories. Each of us brings a unique story and gifts from the Creator. Our stories are about journeys of faith. We walk a path of righteousness. We share our path with all creation. We are related.

Z. Susanne Aikman (Eastern Cherokee) (published in Hofstra 1992)

Beauty Is Before Me

Now talking God, with your feet I walk. I walk with your limbs, I carry forth your body. For me your mind thinks. Your voice speaks for me. Beauty is before me and beauty is behind me. Above and below me hovers the beautiful. I am surrounded by it. I am immersed in it. In my youth, I am aware of it. And in old age I shall walk quietly the beautiful trail.

Navajo prayer tradition by Christian Native American Women for World Day of Prayer 1981

My Spirit Is One with You (prayer for a caregiver)

My spirit is one with you, Creator God. You strengthen me day and night to share my very best with my brothers and sisters. You, whom my people see in all of creation and in all people, show your love for us. Help me to know, like the soaring eagle, the heights of knowledge. From the Four Directions, fill me with the four virtues, fortitude, generosity, respect, and wisdom, so that I will help my people walk the path of understanding and peace.

Lakota prayer tradition

Guiding principles and covenant

The following principles from Native People and The United Methodist Church can be adapted and used as a primer for ministering with and among Native people:

1. We believe in redemption, transformation, and reconciliation; people can change and that is representative of the incarnational witness in the world.
2. We believe in John Wesley's directive to connect social and personal holiness; that advocacy and action, speaking out in the public square, truth-telling in love are intrinsic to who we are as United Methodists.
3. We believe that the intentions and politicization of Christianity distorted the Gospel/Good News for the purpose of colonization and must be decolonized.
4. We affirm that American Indian sovereignty:
    i. Is a historical fact, is significant, and it cannot be disregarded in favor of political expediency
    ii. American Indians have a right to self-govern
    iii. Preserves culture, land, religious expression, and sacred spaces
    iv. Ensures survival—allows for the survival of American Indian people.
5. We need to demythologize and move from fiction to fact in our understanding of American Indians and Indian Country.
6. We affirm the sacredness of humankind:
    i. Affirming all persons as equally valuable in God's sight
    ii. Resources of the world are sacred and deplore practices of exploitation.

7. We reject stereotypes and frames that depict American Indians as less than sacred or in harmful or distorted ways.
8. We observe that there are belief systems of Native American Indians and non-natives and that they do not always have commonality (i.e. "Fair play"/Justice—e.g. land claims, treaties vs. constitutional rights, citizen's rights). (United Methodist Book of Resolutions 2016)

References and further reading

Hofstra, M. (ed.) (1992) *Voices: Native American Hymns and Other Worship Resources.* Nashville, TN: Discipleship Resources.

Mayeda, E.R., Glymour, M.M., Quesenberry, C.P., and Whitmer, R.A. (2016) 'Inequalities in dementia incidence between six racial and ethnic groups over 14 years.' *Alzheimer's & Dementia: The Journal of the Alzheimer's Association 12*, 3, 216–224. Retrieved from www.ncbi.nlm.nih.gov/pubmed/26874595 on November 02, 2018.

SAMHSA (2009) *American Indian and Alaska Native Culture Card: A Guide to Build Cultural Awareness.* Washington, DC: SAMHSA. Retrieved from https://store.samhsa.gov/product/American-Indian-and-Alaska-Native-Culture-Card/SMA084354 on October 10, 2018.

Shabbat Services for Residents with Dementia at Miami Jewish Health

Rabbi Israel de la Piedra (Jewish)

Miami Jewish Health

Miami Jewish Health is one of the largest providers of senior residential and rehabilitation care in South Florida. It was founded over 75 years ago as a small institution called "Miami Jewish Home for the Aged," originally catering mostly to elderly Jewish residents. During its long history the institution has grown and evolved significantly, and now provides residential and medical care services for a large and diverse population of over 700 people in its central location in the city of Miami (in independent living, assisted living, nursing home, rehabilitation, and adult day care settings) and about 250 independent senior residents in its Pembroke Pines, FL campus. The institution is currently embarking on a major expansion project, including the building of the first-of-its-kind village environment for individuals suffering from dementia in the United States, the adoption of a new and pioneering model of care called "EmpathiCare," and a third residential campus.

Notwithstanding its rapid growth and increasing diversity, Miami Jewish Health remains true to the time-honored Jewish values that have guided it since its creation, including honoring the elderly, visiting the sick, and providing true hospitality. These basic principles have led Miami Jewish Health to grow as an institution open to all, where diversity is seen both as a challenge and an opportunity to become a welcoming and inclusive institution providing state-of-the-art care for its residents and patients.

As part of its wholistic approach to the care of the elderly and the ill, Miami Jewish Health provides regular religious services in several different ways. A full-time rabbi acts as director of spiritual care and, in addition to offering pastoral care to residents and patients of all backgrounds, leads weekly and holiday Jewish religious services. Christian religious services are provided regularly by visiting clergy and chaplains. In addition, dedicated volunteers visit residents and patients regularly to offer company and spiritual support.

Jewish religious services at Miami Jewish Health

Several Jewish worship services are offered to the residents and patients of the main campus of Miami Jewish Health every week on Shabbat. These services include a festive "Shabbat Celebration" on Friday afternoons, attended by a large number of both Jewish and non-Jewish residents, including the traditional candle lighting, several elements of Shabbat worship, and live music and singing, and conducted with the help of enthusiastic volunteers. Formal Shabbat services are offered in the campus synagogue on Friday evenings and Saturday mornings in a traditional and egalitarian format (including one monthly Friday evening service conducted in English).[2] Also, a Shabbat service especially designed for the residents of the assisted living facility suffering from dementia takes place every week. In addition to the weekly Shabbat services, all Jewish holidays are celebrated with the appropriate synagogue services, special holiday activities, and celebrations open to all residents.[3]

The Shabbat service for residents with dementia

The Shabbat service for the residents affected by dementia takes place every Friday afternoon in the special floor occupied by the special care unit of the assisted living facility. It is conducted by the rabbi, has a fixed structure of prayer and song, and lasts about 15 minutes. The service is conducted entirely through song; however, instruments such as tambourines and others are purposely not provided to the residents so as to help them identify the service as a worship moment and not just as a musical activity.

When the rabbi arrives, the residents have already been helped by the nursing staff to sit in a semicircle in an open area of their floor. Before the service starts, the rabbi goes around and greets the residents one by one,

2 Synagogue services are beamed by closed-circuit TV to all residents and patients of the main campus of Miami Jewish Health, allowing those who cannot come to the synagogue to follow the services from their apartments and rooms.

3 In addition to these services held in the main campus, a monthly Shabbat service and several holiday celebrations are also offered to the residents of Miami Jewish Health's satellite campus.

and after the service is over the rabbi again goes around to say goodbye personally to every one of the residents.

On average, about 12 to 15 residents attend this weekly service, all of them affected by dementia in varying degrees. About half to two thirds of the residents who attend this service are Jewish and the rest are Christian. All of them speak English, although not all of them are American by birth.

The fixed structure of this short Shabbat service consists of the following eight prayers and songs:

- Shalom Aleichem
- Shabbes, Shabbes
- Hevenu Shalom Aleichem
- Hava Nagila
- Halleluya
- Hineh Ma Tov
- Ose Shalom
- Vene'emar.

The choice of the particular prayers and songs included in this short Shabbat service was guided by three major principles: to elicit a sense of familiarity with the tradition among the Jewish residents; to create a festive atmosphere of celebration and song to mark Shabbat as a special day; and to provide a welcoming environment to the non-Jewish residents who may not be familiar with the prayers and melodies of a Shabbat service. In what follows, we discuss how these three principles were combined to arrive at the particular choice and order of each one of the prayers of this Shabbat service.

The first prayer, "Shalom Aleichem" ("Peace be upon you"), is a melody traditionally sung at the onset of Shabbat, when the family sits down for the Friday evening dinner.[4] The Friday evening meal is the most important family ritual for Shabbat, a time of coming together to celebrate the sacred nature of the day of rest and to enjoy being together with our loved ones and friends. The dinner is preceded by the lighting

4 The Jewish day starts at sundown the day before, and so Shabbat actually starts on Friday evening (and ends on Saturday at sundown).

of the Shabbat candles and other rituals such as the blessing of the children by their parents. The song's words welcome the special angels that accompany a person on Shabbat, asking the angels for their blessing and then sending them away in peace—ideas that may be shared with the residents as the service is starting. Singing Shalom Aleichem helps to evoke warm and reassuring feelings of family and tradition among people who grew up in a Jewish home, while starting the Shabbat service with this song helps to mark the occasion as being unmistakably Shabbat. At the same time, beginning with the upbeat yet traditional melody of Shalom Aleichem helps to set a celebratory tone for the rest of the service.

After singing Shalom Aleichem, the service continues with a Shabbat song in Yiddish, "Shabbes, Shabbes" ("Shabbat, Shabbat"). The Hebrew language is the formal language of prayer in the Jewish tradition (as well as the language of the modern State of Israel); synagogue worship is traditionally conducted in Hebrew, and Jewish people are usually quite familiar with its sounds even if they may not always understand the exact meaning of the Hebrew words they are reciting or singing. Yiddish is a different language, the one brought by the large influx of Jewish immigrants to the United States from Eastern Europe and Russia as their vernacular. Although Yiddish is not usually spoken on a regular basis by the descendants of such immigrants, many people in their eighties and nineties still conserve a strong attachment and familiarity with it—whether because they themselves spoke it when they were young or because they heard their parents speak it. If Hebrew is the formal language of prayer and the language with which to address oneself to God, Yiddish for many of our elders is the Jewish language of the home and the language with which to express their innermost feelings. Including a Yiddish song as the second element of the service is meant to bring up those intimate memories of home, family, and tradition, to complement the more formal memories of Shabbat at the synagogue. Even though Shabbes, Shabbes is not formally prayer, it is a Shabbat song that expresses our hope that we may always be able to celebrate Shabbat and the holidays and to enjoy peace. Singing a song in Yiddish may do more for our elderly Jewish residents than any Hebrew prayer to put them in "Shabbes mode"!

The next two elements of the service, "Hevenu Shalom Aleichem" ("We bring you peace") and "Hava Nagila" ("Let us rejoice"), are two traditional Jewish songs. These are secular compositions rather than prayers, and their inclusion in the service is meant to enhance the Jewish feelings of those attending the service. These songs are universally sung on Jewish occasions, ranging from weddings to Israeli Independence Day celebrations. Singing these secular songs is meant to help even those Jewish residents who have no personal affinity with religious or synagogue services to feel at ease to be joining a Shabbat celebration. The words of these two songs—which refer to peace and to brotherly rejoicing but are sung in Hebrew—may actually matter less than the power of their upbeat and instantly recognizable Jewish melodies as a factor in bringing together Jewish residents of different backgrounds. In addition, and importantly, these Jewish melodies have become part of American culture broadly defined, helping to create a sense of inclusion in the service for the non-Jewish residents, who can enjoy singing or humming along well-known melodies (as opposed to the first two melodies included in the service, with which non-Jewish residents are most likely unfamiliar).

The next element of the service is a prayer that repeats the word "halleluya" in song, over and over again, based on one of the melodies used in synagogue to sing Psalm 150. Only the word "halleluya" is used in this prayer, so as to allow the participants who so desire and are able to sing along to do so. The term "halleluya" is a Hebrew word—meaning "Let us praise God"—but it is universally understood by both Jews and Christians as a key worship word of praise to God. So, all participants in the service, whether Jewish or not, can identify with this song, helping to enhance the sense of the service as inclusive and friendly to all. The meaning of the word "halleluya" also may allow for a brief discussion with the residents of the concept of praising God and its importance.

Following the singing of Halleluya, and reflecting the fact that all residents, Jewish and non-Jewish, seem to be now truly a part of the service, the next prayer, also drawn from the psalms, is "Hineh Ma Tov" ("How good it is [to sit together as brothers]"), a prayer celebrating brotherhood. To make sure that the meaning of the prayer is understood by the residents, it does not hurt to introduce it by saying what the words "hineh ma tov" mean, making reference to the service being held. Although the prayer is in Hebrew, the melody is easy to follow, even if the words may not be; its repetition week after week, like all other prayers in this service, helps the residents identify with it even if they do not understand the Hebrew words.

As the service is now fully back in Hebrew prayer territory, it moves on to another popular Jewish prayer, "Ose Shalom" ("The One who makes peace"). As with the case of Hineh Ma Tov, this prayer is also in Hebrew, but its melody is easy to follow. Jewish worshipers will immediately recognize this prayer and most of them will sing along, while non-Jewish residents will recognize it because its beautiful melody is repeated week after week and because most of them may already be familiar with the word "shalom." The singing of Ose Shalom is usually preceded by a call from the rabbi to the residents to pray for peace—not just peace in a traditional, military sense, but also to pray for personal peace, the peace that comes from enjoying good health, loving family relationships, and tranquility. By offering them hopeful words of peace, the rabbi encourages the residents to pray for their own personal needs as the community as a whole sings Ose Shalom.

The service closes with the singing of "Vene'emar" ("And it is said [that God will be Sovereign over all the world and that on that day God will be one and His name one]"). This is the final line of the prayer "Aleinu" ("It is upon us [to praise the Master of all]"), the prayer that usually closes Jewish prayer services. Singing part of the Aleinu prayer at the end of the service helps the Jewish residents identify what has been going on as a true prayer service, and one which has come to its end. The prayer Aleinu, by the way, is a complex prayer that in its first part stresses the uniqueness of the destiny of the Jewish people and in its second part stresses the ideal unity of humanity. Although the regular Jewish worshiper may not usually be aware of the theological meaning of the different parts of the prayer, in no small measure because the prayer is also in Hebrew, it seems intellectually more honest to end a service attended by Jewish and non-Jewish residents only with that part of the prayer that stresses the unity of mankind rather than with the one that emphasizes the distinctiveness of the Jewish people.

The need for intellectual honesty also explains what some could consider a glaring omission in this Shabbat service: the lack of a recitation of the prayer "Shema Israel" ("Hear O Israel"). The "Shema Israel" prayer is the central declaration of faith of the Jewish people; by reciting it, the worshiper affirms publicly that "the Lord is our God and the Lord is one." Although the literal meaning of the words may not be offensive to non-Jews, the prayer is uniquely Jewish and, for this reason, may not seem to be suitable for a prayer service regularly attended by people of different backgrounds.

The regular Shabbat prayer ends here, but additional prayers and songs can be added at the time of particular holidays, Jewish or otherwise. Every Jewish holiday is associated with certain well-known melodies and one or two of these can easily be added to this short service on the appropriate occasion. Secular holidays also can be marked by singing well-known songs, such as "God Bless America" on the Fourth of July for example. Finally, non-religious songs can be added on occasions such as Christmas as a gesture of goodwill to the non-Jewish residents—who does not like singing "Rudolph the Red-Nosed Reindeer"?

It is important to signal the end of the service. This is done by the rabbi wishing everybody a good Shabbat both in Hebrew and Yiddish after the singing of the last song, whether it is Vene'emar or any special song added for the occasion: "Shabbat Shalom! Gut Shabbes!"

Greeting the residents before and after the service

The prayers and songs described above comprise only one element of the weekly Shabbat service for the residents affected with dementia. In addition, a key component of the service is the personal attention given to the residents by the rabbi. Before the service, the rabbi goes around the room greeting every person present. The rabbi's greetings are intensely personal, drawing heavily on issues that the rabbi knows are important to each resident and include frequent and loving touching gestures. Having thus greeted every one of the residents, the rabbi turns to conducting the service. At the end of the service, the rabbi again goes around the room, saying goodbye to every resident and always in a very personal way.

Even though each one of these personal encounters before and after the service has to be kept very short, they provide the residents with the opportunity to feel appreciated and to bring up any concern that they may have. It is many times surprising how devoting just a few moments of attention to a person can help them bring up an issue that is of importance to them. Just being listened to with empathy goes a long way. The fact that these short interactions with the rabbi are conducted in public is usually not an obstacle for the residents to voice their concerns, and on many occasions these brief personal exchanges allow the rabbi to identify issues that would need to be addressed on a more formal basis with a resident at a later time and with more privacy.

Major lessons learned

Religion in general, and worship in particular, play an important role in the life of people suffering from dementia. Structured and regular religious worship provides them with a channel to express their spiritual needs, connects them to their past and to their traditions, and helps them find a safe haven in the midst of the confusion and the fears brought about by their condition. Although the actual mechanisms by which religion and worship work remain largely unknown, maintaining some aspects of an active religious life has been shown to help maintain a better physical and spiritual health for many of those individuals suffering from dementia.

The short Shabbat service conducted every Friday afternoon in the special care unit of Miami Jewish Health's assisted living facility helps to promote the positive effects of regular worship for its residents affected by dementia. Several reasons combine to make this service an ongoing successful activity. These include: basing the service on song; keeping it short and predictable; keeping a strong emphasis on the personal interaction between the rabbi and each one of the residents as an integral part of service; and last—but not least!—making sure that all practical issues are taken care of to avoid delays and distracting interruptions.

Conducting the service entirely through song has shown to be important for several reasons. Dementia patients seem to maintain an acute sensitivity to song even after other modes of memory stimulation may have waned. By participating in this service, and hearing and singing melodies with which they grew up and which formed an important part of their lives, Jewish residents can successfully bring back reassuring memories of family and tradition. In addition, song gives an opportunity to all the residents attending the service, Jewish and non-Jewish alike, to be active participants. Finally, using song helps to create a cheerful atmosphere, helping to draw the residents in.

It has proven important for the worship service to be kept simple. Simplicity is achieved by ensuring that the service remains short and predictable. A short service allows it to finish before the residents show signs of disorientation, boredom, or confusion. The service is also kept short by the absence of a sermon or of any kind of extended talk; having no sermon helps maintain the rhythm and continuity of the service and promotes the engagement of the residents. However, very short thoughts or simple questions directed to the residents about the prayers or a special occasion being celebrated may be helpful.

The service's predictable nature has been essential to allow the residents to feel that they are entering familiar and unthreatening territory. The fixed and repetitive nature of the songs and prayers used week after week reinforces the sense of familiarity, which in turn helps make the service an anchor for the residents' spirituality while allowing for continued identification with the traditions they grew up with. The predictability of the service is also helped by having a fixed location, a fixed time, and even a fixed prayer leader (in this case, the rabbi). The fixed time of the service brings a sense of order into what is otherwise a life where confusion is ample; indeed, the few times when the time of the service had to be changed, several of the residents were distraught when the usual time arrived and the service did not take place as normally done.

Warm and loving human interaction with the residents attending the service has been one of its key components, helping to ensure the residents' interest in participation. As mentioned above, one of the central parts of the service is the one-on-one interaction that the rabbi has with each one of the residents both before and after the service. In addition, although the service itself does not allow for physical contact between the rabbi and the residents once singing starts, since the rabbi is standing alone in front of the group leading the service, making frequent eye contact with the residents has shown to be very important. This helps to maintain the engagement of the residents with the service and its leader; just as the residents enjoy the personal attention provided by the rabbi's greetings before and after the service, they also appreciate being acknowledged by the rabbi through deliberate eye contact during the service.

Finally, in terms of practical arrangements, there are several points that deserve to be mentioned. Conducting the service in the early afternoon has proven to be a better option than doing so in the morning. Initially the service being discussed was held at 10:30 a.m., but many residents were not ready by that time, were still having breakfast, or were still sleepy. Moving the service to 2:00 p.m. helped to increase attendance significantly, and residents are usually more alert at that time than in the morning. Keeping the number of participants small (no more than 15 at a time) is also essential; a larger number of participants would prevent the rabbi from establishing a personal relationship with each one of them. It is also important to have a strong degree of collaboration with the staff of the special care unit, so that the residents are assembled on time for the service and so that a nursing staff member always remains on hand to deal with any problems that the residents might have during the service.

Conclusion

The weekly Shabbat service for residents suffering from dementia conducted in the special care unit of Miami Jewish Health's assisted living facility has been a success since its inception a few years ago. The service is well liked by the residents, Jewish and non-Jewish alike, and is an important part of their Friday routine. Residents participate by singing or humming along, and most of them tend to remain alert throughout, helped by the service's predictability and reassuring environment. The service gives the Jewish residents an opportunity to mark Shabbat as a special day and to identify with their family and social traditions, while at the same time drawing in the non-Jewish residents based on familiarity with the weekly and upbeat routine. Finally, this service provides the rabbi with an opportunity to greet the residents of the special care unit personally on a regular basis and remains a good vehicle to become aware of any concern that a particular resident may have.

A Buddhist Approach to Connecting with CARE

Rev. Allison Draper, MDiv (Zen Buddhist) and
Rev. Dr. Grace Schireson (Zen Buddhist)

Americans who do not identify with any religious group—the religiously unaffiliated—now account for about one quarter of adults in the U.S., a number that has tripled in size over the last 25 years (Wormald 2015). This presents chaplains who are Buddhist with an interesting opportunity in a culture that is still predominantly Judeo-Christian. While we can minister to Buddhist families, we may also serve many families that like the idea of Buddhism or self-identify as spiritual without a religion. This article will discuss a Buddhist approach to caring for those who identify as Buddhist and also for those who are "Buddhist-friendly"—those who feel spiritual but have no specific religious affiliation or practice.

While a chaplain might come prepared with significant prayers and symbols that would reassure the Buddhist practitioner with dementia, we will need to improvise the approach to caring for the spiritual needs of the areligious, agnostic, or atheistic patient. In any case, we will need to approach with CARE, using these four categories: Context, Assessment, Resources, and Engagement. Context refers to family, spouse, other diagnoses, length of time in facility, and source of referral. Assessment refers to the ability of the dementia patient to communicate verbally and other cognitive skills as evaluated by the family, facility, and the chaplain. Resource refers to the potential supports identified through the assessment tools, conversations, and available communities. Engagement refers to the chaplain's ability to connect with the patient and his/her felt sense of relationship with the patient.

The self-identified Buddhist population in the U.S. is small—0.7 percent (Wormald 2015), dividing into three distinctly different categories of Buddhist practitioners or potential Buddhist observers. Simplistically stated, these categories are: Buddhist Born (BB), Buddhist Converts (BC), and Buddhist Friendly (BF). Buddhist Born (BB) observers primarily come from Asian families and were born into the Buddhist religion. BB celebrate Buddhist holidays with their family and usually have affiliation with a particular sect/temple for holidays, rituals, and family events (e.g. funerals, weddings, memorials).

Buddhist Converts (BC) are individuals who are not necessarily from Buddhist families; instead they have taken up Buddhism as a spiritual practice. BC tend to be affiliated with a particular Buddhist tradition, and may or may not retain some affiliation with the faith tradition of their family of origin. BC tend to meditate or chant and may not be as concerned with Buddhist holidays and ceremonies. While second-generation BC families are now more common in the U.S., this cohort still more closely resembles BC than BB.

The growing body of spiritual but not religious dementia patients may be well served by a Buddhist Friendly (BF) approach. BF share Buddhist values that are environmentally sympathetic and see natural beauty as an expression of a unified energy without theistic connotation. In addition, BF may have adopted a secular form of historically Buddhist practices such as meditation. A 2017 survey found that 18 percent of Americans identify themselves as "spiritual but not religious." Increasingly, the number of individuals who are not affiliated with a religion may not be secular but may be searching for a more personal spirituality that they design to meet their own needs and experience. The dementia patient who is spiritual but not religious may be well served by a chaplain with a BF approach, while those who claim no spiritual affinity might be beyond the chaplain's scope of providing spiritual care. We expect that BF outnumber both BB and BC.

The most commonly observed Buddhist traditions (for BB and BC) are native to Japan, Vietnam, Korea, Southeast Asia, Tibet, or China. The discussion of *all* of these geographically distinct forms of Buddhism is beyond the scope of this article. Therefore, the focus for BB and BC will be only on resources for the two popular forms of Japanese Buddhist worship. These two types of practice, commonly observed in Japan and the U.S., are Jodo Shu or Pure Land (chanting) and Soto Zen (meditation). In addition to presenting simple and basic examples of Buddhist chants, implements, and their community resources, we will also mention ways to connect with BF through poems, quotes, pictures, or objects. Chaplains serving BB, BC, and BF could choose from these simple rituals, chants, and inspiring natural objects as deemed appropriate.

Context

Before planning the approach to spiritual guidance for the dementia patient, the most important considerations and questions are: What was the patient's previous level of functioning with family and community before being referred to the chaplain? What was the basis for the referral to the chaplain or what brought the patient into the institutional setting or home-service which offers this chaplaincy service? This history will help us to make a more thorough assessment of the patient and his/her potential resources. As discussed below, the chaplain should continually gauge and adjust to the patient's ability to engage and recount their spiritual experience. Asking questions that are beyond the patient's cognitive ability may increase anxiety or confusion for the patient. A chaplain will need to question staff, family, friends, religious community, or BF community to understand previous levels of engagement with Buddhism (i.e. BB, BC, or BF) or active avoidance of religion in favor of a non-affiliated spiritual approach.

Important questions

Besides knowing onset and severity of dementia and co-existing medical issues, in order to serve the Buddhist-oriented patient, a chaplain would need to know:

- Did the patient attend regular Buddhist services?
- With which community did s/he practice (including atheistic or agnostic communities)?
- What Buddhist practices did s/he engage in—meditation, mindfulness, contemplation, chanting, Sutra study?
- Did s/he participate in a group that celebrated nature—Sierra Club, hiking, bird watching, or other group?
- Are there any close friends who can visit and share previous worship/nature celebrations?
- After assessment, how do we brief a potential visitor on the patient's current level of functioning and still maintain confidentiality?

Determining the patient's relationship to Buddhist practice

For BB and BC, in both Pure Land and Soto Zen traditions, the community practice is at the center of observances. BB families celebrate Buddhist holidays and also observe Buddhist rituals in the home. The family may have an altar in the home with memorial tablets for the family's ancestors. The family or community (*sangha*) can help the chaplain by identifying the rituals, spiritual implements or symbols, and important holidays. The BF dementia patient may have been part of a hiking group or a community that deemed itself atheistic or agnostic. How current and of what duration are the patient's relationships to those communities?

For BB and BC dementia patients, it would be useful to determine what roles the patient previously played in the community or family practice. For example, a patient may have regularly attended daily meditation or chanting practice, may have attended longer retreats, may have led the chants for the community, or may have cooked for the community. The BF patient may have organized or attended excursions to mountains, the seashore, or bird sanctuaries, or participated in lectures and discussions that explained an agnostic or atheistic view. Exploring the roles that the patient previously enjoyed will help to determine which resources to contact or employ.

Assessment

In the past 20 years, healthcare chaplaincy has increasingly focused on contributing to holistic, person, and family-centered care. This direction comes out of understanding that true care is about meeting a person's unique, holistic needs—physical and spiritual—and in concert with the full support system. As chaplains, our purview is meeting religious, spiritual, emotional, and relational needs. But first, we have to identify those needs—a challenge to assess even for people without memory or cognitive decline. How do we discover the shifting spiritual and emotional needs of persons with dementia? How do we find the way to regularly meet those needs, in conjunction with the family and other caregivers and resources, even as cognitive abilities continue to erode?

Having a simple structure for assessing spiritual background is a great starting point for discussion with the dementia patient (if cognitively appropriate) and with family members or primary caregivers, especially if the person is no longer able to communicate effectively. The format of the spiritual assessment tool is not important, as long as it is easy to remember while conducting a conversation, to allow the chaplain to focus on the person rather than on note-taking.

Chaplains may be familiar with several different models for spiritual assessment used in hospitals, palliative care, and hospice settings. One of the earliest working models, "The Discipline" (VandeCreek and Lucas 2014), advocates for a content-free approach that allows the chaplain to make a context-appropriate response. This model, and most spiritual assessment approaches now in use, asks the chaplain to have an intentional conversation with the care recipient to assess their needs, hopes, or desired outcome, and current level of support. From this conversation, the chaplain creates a profile of the care recipient's sense of sacred, meaning, hope, and community, envisions an approach to spiritual care, and articulates how this integrates with the rest of the support system. Of course, the chaplain's warm presence and active listening skills to connect with the patient's narrative, or their story as told by close family and friends, are the starting point and guide throughout.

The FACT assessment tool is commonly used by professional chaplains in acute care settings. The FACT acronym is a way to recall categories to prompt further discussion in friendly conversation. After this discussion, the chaplain can jot notes and fill out the assessment. Because the FACT spiritual assessment tool is short, easy, and flexible, it can be used effectively with people with dementia or their caregivers.

F—Facts about the dementia patient's situation, including: Facility (medical and cognitive); Feelings; Family; Faith (Religious Tradition, Beliefs, Spiritual Practices); Fun

A—Active (and/or Availability vs. Anxiety)

C—Coping (and/or Comfort); Conflict (and/or Concern)

T—Treatment Plan

The "A" in the FACT assessment is about discerning which of the "F" category resources are available, immediately or on request, versus those which are absent in the person's support network. The "C" is about assessing how well the person and family are coping. A simple way to determine "T" treatments is for the chaplain to look for the biggest gaps, where an important "F" category is not a source of comfort, but rather the patient or family is feeling some concern or conflict about it.

FACT can be adapted to allow for inquiry around the complex interactions among religious, spiritual, cultural, and family-related factors; this is especially critical for those who are outside the predominantly Judeo-Christian culture. Religious values and practices are deeply embedded within societies, and underpin personal feelings of identity, belonging, and worth. In working with memory-compromised persons, it's important to pay particular care to the expressed feelings and memories around religious affiliation (or lack thereof) and its intersection with a sense of spirituality, belonging, and support.

From a Buddhist perspective, respectful listening with open presence is an important mechanism for assessing needs, since attuning to inner experience is a central aspect of the religion. Particular attention is important around the individual's Buddhist identity, and how this relates to family, friends, community, and other elements of their support system. Born Buddhists may have access to childhood memories that positively associate religious, cultural, and family traditions. Whether active in the religious community or not, BBs may rely on the local temple for important emotional connections, in their native language—a role that assimilated family members may or may not be able to provide. Buddhist Converts may also depend on a local Buddhist community to meet the emotional and spiritual needs that family cannot. BCs' beliefs and religious practices may be in contrast to, or even in conflict with, those of their family of origin.

Whether because of immigration or because of an intentional spiritual choice, Buddhists in the United States may feel a heightened sense of separation from the familial, cultural, and religious traditions of their upbringing, adding complexity to the spiritual care of those suffering from memory impairment. The chaplain's most important role may be an ongoing conversation, attuning to and assessing the shifting territory of the care recipient's experience, and helping to identify appropriate resources along the way.

Resources

Here is a checklist for planning purposes and for contacting potential resources.

Buddhist spiritual care checklist

- ☐ BB, BC: Previous temple/community contacts
  - ☐ Favorite chants
  - ☐ Favorite/familiar objects
  - ☐ Family/home altar
- ☐ BF: Previous solo or group activities
  - ☐ Group contacts
  - ☐ Group activities
  - ☐ Group philosophies/favorite authors
- ☐ BB, BC, BF: Family supportive of patient's spiritual inclination?

Dementia patients are invariably in a long, slow decline toward end of life. Assessing and resourcing are an ongoing process—perhaps over several years, if the chaplain has been brought in early in the dementia's onset. Even if the dementia patient is not receiving palliative or hospice care, at some level, the patient and family may sense the downward trajectory. No matter what the faith background, the dementia diagnosis itself can cause trepidation, along with existential or spiritual distress.

Patients may worry about their independence and becoming a burden. Families and friends may worry about their ability to cope and provide the necessary financial, physical, and emotional support. Yet, because of the slow decline and uncertainty of capabilities along the way, this distress may be lurking under the surface. Buddhism's culture of equanimity, which places high value on appearing calm and self-controlled under any circumstances, could cause the dementia patient or family caregivers to not show or share difficult feelings, and not accept help until late stages of the dementia process.

In resourcing faith support for Buddhists, the chaplain should bear in mind that needs may differ greatly based on the degree to which religious practices are intertwined with the dementia patient's culture and daily living arrangements. For example, BBs may rely on a local temple community for social and cultural support, and to celebrate Buddhist holidays, but be less engaged in everyday formal practices. Conversely, BCs may look to their Buddhist community for formal ongoing practice support, while getting social and cultural support from family and friends who are not Buddhist. Chanting and/or meditation may be a daily at-home practice for many Buddhists of either type, as well as for many who are BF.

In our experience, meditation and simple chants can help quell anxious feelings in the moment and, if repeated regularly, can move a person toward acceptance and integration of difficult life-altering experiences. A growing body of brain research suggests that mindfulness practices can slow, or possibly counteract, cognitive decline (Gard, Hölzel, and Lazar 2014). We've also seen that meditation could increase anxiety in the cognitively impaired or anxious patient, even if they have had a well-established practice before. This is why, no matter what the research suggests, nothing can substitute for the chaplain's eyes and ears!

The chaplain may contact a local temple willing to send monks or community members to chant or meditate with a patient. If the chaplain is comfortable and invited to do so, she may also offer to chant or meditate with the patient (see the end of the article for basic chants for Pure Land and Soto Zen). It's important to take the lead from the patient, their family, and their temple about appropriateness and preferences. One feature of dementia is the need to stick to familiar routines. For example, a recorded chant from the patient's particular Buddhist sect played on an iPhone might be appropriate and comforting. Some traditional Asian Buddhist temples sell inexpensive "Buddha boxes," which play chants on a continuous loop.

In our experience, the intensity of needs and level of resources increase sharply as the patient becomes more fully dependent and nears end-of-life. The support system, which many have been adequately managing for some time, can quickly become overwhelmed with the demands of round-the-clock caring, especially during peak periods in the early evening if the patient is prone to "sundowning." Helping the household or care facility establish and maintain the patient's familiar Buddhist practices—chanting, meditation, or both—can be a very important resource for everyone to rely on during the end-stage. Many chants are reassuring even to non-Buddhist family and friends through comforting, harmonious sound and with words about taking refuge or reaching the end of the cycle of suffering.

A chaplain for Buddhist dementia patients can check into national Buddhist associations for local members who may be willing to help if there are no familiar contacts. For the Soto Zen example, one can find online a Soto Zen Buddhist Association (BC), an Association of Soto Zen Buddhists (BB and BC), and an Association of Secular Buddhists (BF).

For the Pure Land Buddhist examples, there is the Shin Dharma Net, the Institute of Buddhist Studies, and Buddhist Churches of America. These organizations can redirect to their local affiliates.

Engagement

Dementia patients are usually referred to an in-home palliative care or hospice team, or placed in a care facility after loss of function has made daily activities difficult, unsafe, or impossible to complete. With these losses in mind, conversation with the patient on spirituality may not be possible. However, it may be possible to provide an appropriate spiritual or religious engagement in which the patient can participate (actively or passively) by consulting designated resources or a chaplain or another well-trained spiritual director.

A foundational approach to helping patients was developed by Carl Rogers (1980). Rogers taught that for a person to be helped, one needs an environment that provides him/her with: a) genuineness (openness and self-disclosure), b) acceptance (being seen with unconditional positive regard), and c) empathy (being listened to and understood). The chaplain for a Buddhist-affiliated dementia patient needs to create a field of acceptance. This is why it is so important to be prepared for, and to prepare other resources for, the dementia patient's actual abilities—even as they may decline.

The chaplain is not there to "improve" the patient's cognition or create new spiritual content. The chaplain is there to offer a connection to the patient's pre-existing spiritual world. This connection depends on proceeding with awareness and overt care and kindness. In Buddhism, we might refer to this mind state as cultivating the empty field. By this we mean that we move our expectations and feelings to one side and actively create space within which the patient may join us. If we learn to do this, we can watch our own sense of connection to the patient on each visit. Self-observation is key to adjusting to the patient's needs. During the time we are with the patient, we must be guided by his/her own receptivity to our offering and our connection. Buddhists describe this process as "reaching for a pillow in the dark" (X. and Cleary 2005, p.229). We do not know where it is, but we know it when we feel it.

Someone offering a spiritual connection to a patient would do well to engage their own spiritual centering—whether it be prayer, meditation, or chanting—prior to each meeting with the patient. From an open-minded, judgment-free view, one can more readily experience the patient's level of well-being or anxiety. What is the dementia patient experiencing? One can quietly observe non-verbal cues: changing facial expression, respiration rate, skin tone, voluntary and involuntary hand gestures, and tone of voice. If the patient is verbal and can converse, we should still note the patient's non-verbal cues even as we engage in conversation. If the patient is non-verbal, we can attempt to synchronize our breathing with him/her. This connection may help the chaplain to be more centered and may offer a deep connection to the patient.

When offering support to a Buddhist dementia patient, we will probably not have the same ubiquitous tools or symbols common in our Judeo-Christian culture. If the BB or BC patient has engaged with a specific community, we can make use of familiar chanting, bell ringing, Buddha statues, or incense familiar to the patient. If the patient is BF, we may use photographs of animals, forest, sky, or ocean to share a sense of profound unity with the patient through imagery and accompanying poetry. An important Soto Zen poem talks about the reflection of this profound unity and interconnection of all as one as "The moon in a dewdrop" (Dogen and Tanahashi 1995).

Conclusion

A Buddhist approach to chaplaincy with dementia patients may work well for Buddhist Converts (BC), Buddhist Born (BB), and a growing number of non-religious-affiliated Buddhist Friendly (BF) patients. Providing religious, spiritual, emotional, and relational support to dementia patients who have lost significant daily functions and cognitive ability is challenging in any circumstance. For those who are outside the predominantly Judeo-Christian culture, the challenges and the need for spiritual support may be even greater. As with those who affiliate with any established religious tradition and community, Buddhist-affiliated dementia patients may feel reassured by the ministering of familiar practices, prayers, and symbols. But because this population's spiritual background and shifting landscape is more complex, and the need to assess and connect without the explicit input of the patient him/herself, the chaplain's work requires improvisation. We offer CARE (Context, Assessment, Resources, and Engagement) as a mindful approach to working with Buddhist and Buddhist-friendly dementia patients.

The chaplain learning how to help a Buddhist dementia patient will need to explore unknown territory. A Zen founder in America, Shunryu Suzuki, described the potential of the beginner's mind. He often said that there were many possibilities in a beginner's mind, but few in the expert's mind. With no path in mind, one must first study the different ways (Context) Buddhist members participate in practice to gather the fundamentals of the patient's spirituality. In the Assessment phase, the chaplain is interested in the patient's life while treading lightly when gathering data. Holding a spirit of inquiry is also important in gathering Resources, contacting and recruiting the patient's connections. Finally, for Engagement, a chaplain will practice being centered and open with the patient. An old Zen Buddhist expression teaches that not knowing is most intimate. If we think we know, we have closed ourselves off from the relationship. By not knowing, we feel our way, breath by breath.

Chants

For Soto Zen

Refuges (BB)

Namu kie butsu
Namu kie ho
Namu kie so

Refuges (BC)

I take refuge in the Buddha
I take refuge in the Dharma
I take refuge in the Sangha

Meditation Robe Chant (BC)

Great robe of liberation
Field far beyond form and emptiness
Wearing the Tathagatas teaching
Saving all beings

For Pure Land (Jodo Shu) (BB, BC)

Namu amida butsu
Namu myoho renge kyo

Objects

For Soto Zen (BB, BC)

Bells, juzu beads, Buddha statues

For Pure Land

Juzu beads, recorded chants

Bibliography

X. and Cleary, T.F. (2005) *Book of Serenity: One Hundred Zen Dialogues*. Boston, MA: Shambhala.

Dogen, E. (auth.) and Tanahashi, K. (ed.) (1995) *Moon in a Dewdrop*. San Francisco, CA: North Point Press.

Gard, T., Hölzel, B.K., and Lazar, S.W. (2014) 'The potential effects of meditation on age-related cognitive decline: A systematic review.' *Annals of the New York Academy of Sciences 1307*, 1, 89–103.

Larocca-Pitts, M.A. (2009) 'FACT: Taking a spiritual history in a clinical setting.' *Journal of Health Care Chaplaincy 15*, 1, 1–12.

Lipka, M. and Gecewicz, C. (2017) 'More Americans now say they're spiritual but not religious.' Retrieved from www.pewresearch.org/fact-tank/2017/09/06/more-americans-now-say-theyre-spiritual-but-not-religious on November 02, 2018.

Raney, A., Cox, D., and Jones, R. (2017) 'Searching for spirituality in the U.S.: A new look at the spiritual but not religious.' Retrieved from https://www.prri.org/research/religiosity-and-spirituality-in-america on February 13, 2018.

Rogers, C.R. (1980) *Way of Being*. Boston, MA: Houghton.

Tanahashi, K. and Nagase, M. (2015) *Zen Chants: Thirty-Five Essential Texts with Commentary*. Boston, MA: Shambhala.

VandeCreek, L. and Lucas, A.M. (2014) *The Discipline for Pastoral Care Giving Foundations for Outcome Oriented Chaplaincy*. Hoboken, NJ: Taylor and Francis.

Wormald, B. (2015) 'America's changing religious landscape.' Retrieved from www.pewforum.org/2015/05/12/americas-changing-religious-landscape on February 11, 2018.

Memory Care and Shabbat

Dr. Andrea (Yonina) K. Foster (Jewish)

I would ring the doorbell and await a staff member beeping me in. A short time later I'd sing several rounds of "Yadaidaidaidai...," a wordless melody, with Cohen-Rosen House residents, and follow it with "Ivdu et Hashem," "Serve God with Gladness." Thus would begin Shabbat in Memory Care at Charles E. Smith Life Communities in Rockville, Maryland, where I facilitated afternoon services with residents, welcoming in the Jewish day of rest, until I moved to Buffalo, New York, after my husband's death.

Imagine it is Friday afternoon, 4:00 p.m., when I am meeting residents in their living room. They are alert, dozing, asleep. Some smile, talk, laugh. They also might sing, shake a tambourine, or beat a small drum. I "meet them where they are" as we said in Clinical Pastoral Education studies. Moments here at Cohen-Rosen are holy in a way not always easy to explain. Some are most difficult, others joyful.

The residents, according to Cohen-Rosen House Manager Dale Zazanis, have Alzheimer's disease with related dementias. The dementias include Lewy Body, Pick's disease, frontotemporal, and vascular dementia.[5] These are progressive dementias and, she told me, "we adjust our person-centered care to the needs of the resident during each phase of their decline. In addition, Parkinson's disease is commonly listed under the 'dementia umbrella' as people with Parkinson's develop dementia-related symptoms." The caregivers, Ms. Zazanis continued, "are trained to approach all confusion with our residents using 'Validation Therapy,' the common form of communication used today to assist in keeping residents calm."

These residents, in all phases of Alzheimer's and related dementias, men and women, sit in an inner ring of the room facing the fireplace. In this way residents can see and interact with each other in whatever manner they are able to. Residents sit on chairs and couches, interspersed with those in wheelchairs. Walkers are nearby or set off to the side. Cushions keep some people upright and comfortable in their seats.

5 The Cohen-Rosen House Manager, Dale Zazanis, kindly communicated this information to me via an e-mail, November 10, 2017.

Residents also are seated in an outer ring of seats near windows, where comfortable chairs are arranged. There is a walkway between the outer ring and those nearer to where I sit in front of the fireplace. The staff assist, keeping a watchful eye when a resident calls out, leans over too far, or needs to get up. One staff member carries a basket of small rhythm instruments and offers them around the room.

The cart with the juice and the challah, braided bread, special for Shabbat, is readily available for the time of the blessings later on. If I remember, I check the batteries in the candles I'll switch on soon after we begin to settle in to initiate the Sabbath, even though the official time for the candles is much later. I make sure my prayer binder is ready on the music stand, guitar tuned, and Chatter Vox is on and working so I have a personal audio system. Those who are hard of hearing can hear me. I can speak in a normal voice.

I settle at the piano bench brought in front to complete the circle. The bench allows me to slide on and off easily to get up with my 3/4 size guitar and move among the residents to sing, ask questions, and even dance a little. The entire time I'm preparing and looking around, I greet the residents who have become my family, people I've seen in stages of stability and decline. Before I officially begin, I go to the restroom and wash my hands. Sometimes I'll reach out to a resident, shake hands, place my arm on a shoulder as I pass. It's always important to have hands washed before I begin, for the residents' health and my own.

"Hello, Jan, it's good to see you. And Herb, you, too. Lovely day today. Bright sun in here! I'm back for Shabbat. Traffic was the usual. I know some of you know what that's like around here. How has your day been?" I ask. Even if I don't say someone's name, I look around the room and acknowledge everyone the best I can with a smile, a nod. I might even blow a kiss. Frequently, grown children of the residents are here. This Friday afternoon it's a sisterhood. Sons come, too, more often on the weekends when I've been there for programs. Grandchildren also visit, and are welcomed by all.

From the opening nigun, a wordless Jewish melody, residents join in, play some instruments, and sing if they are able and choose to. Some simply smile. This afternoon I move on to "Zol Zayn Shabbas." It means "Let it be Shabbas," one resident reminds me. She grew up speaking Yiddish in her home. Several neighbors in Cohen-Rosen speak some Yiddish, one Polish, a Holocaust survivor. She is unable to easily communicate anymore, so we don't know her experiences in

World War II. We can join in with "Yababababababa bam bam bam," and ponder if there is any healing in the song and our being together.

Soon after we begin the songs, I put my guitar down, turn around to the fireplace mantle, and flip the switch so the candles flicker. There are two of them, the traditional number used for Shabbat in some homes. I walk around behind the couch furthest from the fireplace reminding housemates that these candles are battery operated, that there is no real flame or fire threat. We chant the candle blessing and I suggest they move their arms if able to to bring in the Shabbat light, bring in family not here, friends, whomever they want to recall. And we take in the breath of Shabbat while beginning to hum the tune for "Shalom Aleichem," "Peace Be with You," a traditional Shabbat song about welcoming the Sabbath angels.

"Shalom Aleichem" is a favorite and many are able to sing either the tune or the words. As we welcome the angels, singing in Hebrew, as they bring us peace, enter in peace, bless us, then leave, perhaps to move onto the next house for Shabbat, I invite everyone to think of the angels in the room, and those unseen. I mention adult children who are there and staff whose names I do my best to know. I walk back around and fill the juice glasses so that a short time later I can be ready for the blessing over the "wine."

I have a prayer booklet a previous Shabbat leader used. However, the residents' hands are free of any booklets. This allows them to participate in a different way. No booklets falling out of hands and struggles to retrieve them and follow pages they can barely read or hold for long. And I allow fluidity for myself to bring in tunes the community likes, such as "Tumbalalaika," a waltz melody which invites movement and an opportunity to take someone's hand and "dance," with them. "Dodi Li," "My Beloved is Mine," with several different tunes available, or "Az De Rebbe Est," an upbeat song about a Rabbi and his students. "Heiveinu Shalom," "Peace Be upon You," is one most people know, either to sing, to hum, or play the rhythm instruments to. "V'shamru," about the Jewish people guarding the Sabbath, is another often included. It is traditional and one most residents know. Include songs the residents can sing. Offer songs and tunes they enjoy. Ask them to sing for you if you have a question. You'll know for sure what they know when people join you.

All along the way, I gauge the community, the residents, and how long we have before they are accompanied into their dining room for dinner. I keep a watch on the time as I allow for a flow of time in this experience.

I may take longer one week with a song and have little conversations with residents or family members, including all in the sharings of the week. Sometimes I ask questions, wondering who, if anyone, will respond. Sometimes it's a visitor who shares a story about their parent or relative. That adds a special element to our afternoon.

We move into the wine blessing and sometimes a staff member assists in passing out cups with juice for tasting, rather than an overflowing cup. Family members help also. As residents receive their juice, I decide how that afternoon I will offer "To Life, to Life, L'chayim," from the well-known musical *Fiddler on the Roof.* I laminated 8x10 cards, or pages with words, illustrations, and pictures, from the song. It's comical and funny as I stand, or sit, to share the pictures while we sing. The visuals add a dimension to our Shabbat experience with humor and delight. I do my best to hold each card up and show them around. Laughing is so important here, essential in this experience because there is much that is not funny as one's parent, sibling, spouse loses the familiar self one has come to know and becomes someone almost unrecognizable.

We move to singing "L'cha Dodi," "Come My Beloved," a song that welcomes the Sabbath bride. Many tunes prompt different moods and movement possibilities. There is a wonderful image initiated by the Jewish mystics of Safed, Israel, in the 1600s that Shabbat is a wedding between the Jewish people and God. Shabbat, therefore, is a joyful time, yet with meditative moments. For the last verse I stand and face west, or a door, to welcome the Sabbath. Most in the room are seated. Sometimes I dance among the chairs on the chorus.

While it is wonderful to be able to do a religious service for the community, in this setting I modify it and give "tastes," bits and pieces, following the flow of tradition, mostly flowing from one song to another. At times, though not every week, I'll give a minute or two of silence for an Amidah, a standing prayer, in the synagogue. The quiet that arises is awe-inspiring as it pervades the atmosphere when the opportunity is introduced in this setting. We end these moments with the traditional "Oseh Shalom," "The One who Makes Peace." Always, most join in.

As we near the end of our afternoon Shabbat service, I am reminded by a family member to do the blessing for the challah. Sometimes I forget. They are kind to me then, as always. As with the other blessings, for the candles, and the wine, I do this one in Hebrew. I stand among the residents in the inner circle. Then I translate so everyone is on the same "page." We are thankful for the grain of the earth provided... If I am passing out challah, I put gloves on before I start. Otherwise, a staff or family member might do the same to help out. I rarely ask. Often, others ask if they can help. I make sure to walk to the outer circle also, to include everyone near the windows even if they seem to be asleep. How often someone seems asleep and I witness the toe-tapping or nod of the head.

We finish with "Adon Olam," "Ruler of the World." The daughter of a resident requested a particular tune and we go with that one. I have the words and some residents know all the verses and join in, especially with the chorus. Sometimes this is one sung with gusto by those who are hardly heard during the rest of the service.

I have a singable tune for a version of the priestly blessing, with words in English, and I offer it near the end. We take a breath and wish each other Good Shabbat and sing another familiar tune, "Shabbat Shalom" together, blowing a kiss to one another during one of the verses. As I finish up, I put away my guitar and music and converse with those nearby. I stand to leave with my wheeled suitcase behind me, my guitar now slung on my back. One resident asks if I have a ride home and I reassure her I do. Neighbors are being escorted, wheeled, assisted, into the dining room on the other side of the fireplace as I wheel my own suitcase to the doorway and wait to be beeped out. I wish everyone a "Good Shabbat" and exit with a daughter of one of the residents.

Note: Names of residents are changed.

I studied two units of Clinical Pastoral Education (CPE) with Rabbi Jim Michaels, Supervisor, while in ALEPH Seminary as a rabbinic student. During CPE I understood something about myself, that when I showed up I made a difference. I created *Musical Memories*, and subsequently withdrew from my rabbinic studies, a life-long dream, to instead make a difference by showing up with music and conversation, and an intuitive ear for listening and allowing healing at whatever level it might occur.

Seeing the Spirit through Dementia

A Sikh Dharma Perspective

Amar Atma Singh Khalsa, Dharma Singh Khalsa, MD, Ek Ong Kaar Kaur Khalsa Michaud, Kirti Kaur Khalsa, Sarb Nam Kaur Khalsa, and Sarb Sarang Kaur Khalsa (Sikh Dharma)

The Identity of the Heart

by Ek Ong Kaar Kaur Khalsa Michaud

In the Sikh tradition, we say that the Divine lives in the heart of every person as Light. This Light of the Spirit neither takes birth nor dies. It does not come and it does not go. It is uniquely manifested in each individual being and is also inseparably connected to the One Divine Consciousness that oversees and guides the entire Creation. Siri Singh Sahib Bhai Sahib Harbhajan Singh Khalsa Yogiji expressed this so beautifully in saying:

> One day perhaps you'll wake up from the long sleep of the night of the shadow. You'll wake up to the fact that there was no prayer for you. There was no God for you. There was nothing for you except you, and you were the prayer; you were the God and you were the Self. (Chief Religious Authority for Sikh Dharma in the Western Hemisphere, December 7, 1995)

One common phrase for death in the Sikh tradition is "dropping the robe of the body." A Sikh believes that the body clothes the Divine Light. When the clothing gets worn out, the Light simply discards it. We are also not our mind. In Sikh (and yogic) tradition, the mind is considered a separate entity from the Spirit. The mind is considered to be the servant of the Light, not the master, and not the "real" identity of a person. A person's thoughts, ideas, memories, opinions, and preferences (things that we often consider as our identity) are actually not the True Being at all; they are servants of the Soul. When the body-clothing is discarded at the time of death and physical release, the servant-mind also dissolves, while the Light Consciousness (Soul) continues on.

One of the challenges in today's world is that technological advances have given our physical bodies much more longevity than known in recorded history. Unfortunately, our minds do not always experience the same vitality as our bodies as we move into middle and old age. Alzheimer's disease and related dementias as well as mental illness have become a very real part of family and community life. One of the challenges we face as ministers is how to minister to the Light of the person in these situations, rather than to their minds.

In the Sikh community where I have lived for many years in Northern New Mexico, I have seen many people in the last few years drop the robes of their bodies. The majority of these people had serious physical ailments, such as cancer, which slowly or quickly unstitched their body-clothing, leading to their transition from the earthly realm.

For these folks, we would come together as a community each night, at the person's home, as their physical vitality declined, and we would sing together. Singing sacred music is an integral aspect of the Sikh tradition. Singing each night in the home of the dying community member gave spiritual and social support to the family, as well as spiritual connection and support to the person whose body was becoming more worn out each day.

In essence, we took some of the most powerful aspects of our worship services—the singing of sacred music and the reading of sacred prayers—and brought them to the living room of the home where support was needed.

Through this process, the community member who was dying had a chance to share some of his or her experiences of the death process with those gathered, if they chose. This became a beautiful learning experience and source of bonding for everyone present. It made the final days of the person's life a true celebration, sharing uplifting times of laughter, as well as sadness; sharing togetherness and support as well as separation and loss.

When it comes to dementia, walking with the person affected often becomes even more challenging. Our idea of who that person is, along with trying to learn how to communicate with them and relate to them, is radically altered. We recognize the body-robe. But the servant-mind undergoes a profound transformation. Each case of dementia is different, and the process dementia follows is unpredictable. So how can one minister in this type of situation?

There was one member of our community who developed a form of dementia. It happened slowly, over years. The process of diagnosis was exhausting for his family. The hope of treatment proved elusive. The burden on the family was profound, and at the time it appeared that there was very little that our community could do to help.

Over time, this particular community member was no longer recognizable. He was like a child in a man's body. Insistent about doing what he wanted, he would sneak away, and walk for miles on his own when no one would take him where he wanted to go.

We all became aware of what was happening. His wife asked for everyone to keep an eye out, in case he went wandering on his own. Eventually, the family decided to place him in a facility with caregivers who had the skills to handle the demands of what was happening. Shortly after being sent to the facility, he dropped the robe of his physical body and left the earth plane.

Dementia offers a unique challenge because it is the servant-mind that gets exhausted before the body-robe is worn out. There are drugs, facilities, and family and professional care partners who can help. But the dilemma is that, even if the body is healthy, dementia takes a person into a death process somewhat or entirely disconnected from the life he or she had previously lived.

So, what would happen if we viewed dementia as part of the Spirit's decision about how to exit the earth plane?

In a spiritual sense, dementia could be seen as being connected to the Spirit's decision that it needs to sever earthly attachments before dropping the physical body. The work of ministry in this situation might be to acknowledge the Spirit's need to dissolve mental and emotional attachments first, before physical death can happen. Ministering in these situations focuses on supporting the family in the process of letting go of the person's identity, and helping them to connect with their loved one's Spirit. The Spirit Intelligence still exists in the heart of the dementia sufferer. And dementia asks that we find a way to communicate with, hear, understand, and serve that Spirit.

There are many sacred Sikh songs/hymns that speak directly to the mind about the need to let go of earthly attachment in order to be attached only to God. Singing these particular hymns with the family and for the person with dementia can be very helpful and comforting.

Gurmukhi, the Divine language of the Sikh Masters, was created to deeply penetrate the spirit/psyche in order to heal deeply, even when the meaning of the words is not understood. *Gurmukhi* is a language designed to elevate the mind, body, and spirit. Playing the Sikh *shabds* (hymns) and mantras on a continuous-playing music device brings a healing vibration to the individual and family.

The religion of Sikhism was born in India and draws on ancient spiritual teachings from the East. In this modern era, in the West, these Sikh traditions have been intertwined with age-old yogic traditions, through the teachings of Yogi Bhajan (aka "the Siri Singh Sahib"), who brought these yogic gems to seekers in the West in the late 1960s, along with exposing his students to the path of Sikhism. Many individuals practice Sikhism and yogic technology.

Dr. Dharma Singh and his wife Kirti Kaur are both ordained Ministers of Sikh Dharma in the West and students of Yogi Bhajan. In 2003, they founded the Alzheimer's Research and Prevention Foundation (ARPF).[6] Their organization funds research on the cognitive effects of an ancient, yet simple, yogic meditation taught by Yogi Bhajan, Kirtan Kriya (see the next page). This meditation practice has been shown to offer improvements in numerous measures of memory and cognition, as measured by standard neuro-cognitive assessments, as well as a decrease in inflammatory markers, improvement in genetic health, and important traits of quality of life, such as clarity of purpose and spiritual well-being, both in the patient and the care partner. This body of work has been published in over 20 scientific papers since then.

6 www.alzheimersprevention.org

ALZHEIMER'S RESEARCH & PREVENTION FOUNDATION™
a 501(c)(3) charitable organization

Kirtan Kriya Yoga Meditation

The Alzheimer's Research & Prevention Foundation has assembled this information on the Kirtan Kriya singing exercise for medical professionals, the public, caregivers, the media, and anyone interested in improving their brain function and improving memory loss.

Kirtan Kriya exercise utilizes the primal sounds—and is meant to be practiced for greater attention, concentration, focus, improved short-term memory, and better mood. The primal sounds consist of:

- Saa Taa Naa Maa
- The sounds are chanted repeatedly and in order (i.e. Saa Taa Naa Maa). They come from the mantra "Sat Nam," which means "my true essence."

Kirtan Kriya Instructions

If you would like to practice the Kirtan Kriya singing exercise, here are the basic steps:

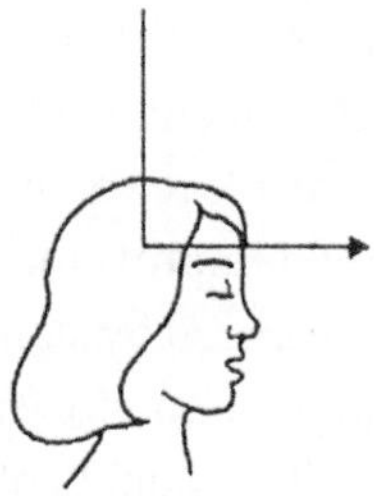

- Repeat the *Saa Taa Naa Maa* sounds (or mantra) while sitting with your spine straight.
- If possible, your focus of concentration is the L form (see illustration at right), while your eyes are closed. With each syllable, imagine the sound flowing in through the top of your head and out the middle of your forehead (your third eye point).
- For two minutes, sing in your normal voice.
- For the next two minutes, sing in a whisper.
- For the next four minutes, say the sound silently to yourself.
- Then reverse the order, whispering for two minutes, and then out loud for two minutes, for a total of twelve minutes.
- To come out of the exercise, inhale very deeply, stretch your hands above your head, and then bring them down slowly in a sweeping motion as you exhale.
- The finger positions are very important in this kriya (see illustration below).
- On *Saa*, touch the index fingers of each hand to your thumbs.
- On *Taa*, touch your middle fingers to your thumbs.
- On *Naa*, touch your ring fingers to your thumbs.
- On *Maa*, touch your little fingers to your thumbs.

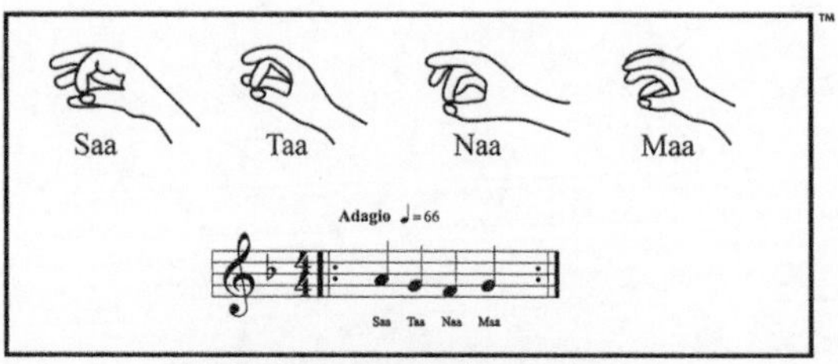

You can order your own copy of Kirtan Kriya at www.alzheimersprevention.org

info@alzheimersprevention.org

Depending on the state of the dementia, and how active a person is, there is also an approach to prayer called Celestial Communication. This technology comes from the Kundalini Yoga tradition as taught by Yogi Bhajan and has the ability to relieve stress for both the person with dementia and their families. Through Celestial Communication, we sing very simple, uplifting songs, with expressive hand gestures that engage the Spirit in a kinesthetic experience of worship that brings joy and openness to the heart through prayerful play, or playful prayer.[7]

When it comes to dementia, I believe we need to expand our idea of worship to include *deep listening*. The persons with dementia and their families need support during the decline and passing of a person with dementia. Listening is tremendously powerful. We do not often think of listening to each other as a form of worship. And yet, if the Divine truly lives in the heart of our Self and of each other, what higher form of worship can there be?

If we sit and simply listen—to the pain, to the confusion, to the uncertainty—the burden to everyone can often be lifted. Finding the time and space to be present while the process of a loved one's dementia unfolds is one form of ministering.

Last but not least, listening to the person with dementia can be a powerful experience. Tune into the Spirit that is asking to communicate, crying to be heard. I have a personal experience of this need. One day, I saw the man in our community with dementia out wandering alone. I did my best to connect with him. He was walking along the side of the road, and I finally coaxed him into my car. He was clearly trying to get somewhere, looking for a place that he could not explain or direct me to find. He definitely did not want to go back to his house. He felt frustrated with everyone trying to keep him at home.

I did my best to listen to him and to respect what he felt. I wanted to hear what he was saying. Somehow, by entering into his perception as best I could, he let me drive him back to his house.

Looking back on this event, I wonder if his Spirit was saying: "It's time for me to move on. That house where you keep taking me is no longer my home. I have to go. I have to get to this other place. Help me get there or let me go. I feel frustrated and angry with all of the people getting in my way."

7 For more information, visit www.super-health.net/celestial-communication-therapy

Another form of ministering is found in organizing earthly support, whether by arranging for meals to be prepared by community members, contributing financial resources, or scheduling a massage for a care partner. The families of those with dementia always need extra support. Often, they hardly have time to figure out what they need. Taking the time to arrange and offer support on the earth plane can also create ease and comfort for the person with dementia, and for their families. Community support is key and profound at these times.

In the decades ahead, as dementia affects more and more people and families, when it comes to worship and ministry I would offer this question for us to consider: "Can we view dementia as part of the Spirit's journey? Can we learn to listen to the person with dementia, and relate to that person as a Spirit longing to tell us what the next leg of this journey can be?"

The mystical process of the Divine

by Ek Ong Kaar Kaur Khalsa Michaud

The Divine Spirit is in each person, shining even through illness, loss, diminishment, and transformation. When talking about Divinity, sometimes we look outside of ourselves to discuss and define God. The Creator becomes, through our own conversations, everything a human is *not*. All-powerful. All-knowing. All-seeing. All-loving. All-kindness. It is as if we humans have taken certain experiences that give us a sense of comfort, that give us a sense of security on the earth; and projected their most perfect and continual expression on a Divine Being who can do and be everything we would most like to be, but aren't.

Guru Nanak gave the Mool Mantra as the essence of the Sikh teachings. Recently, while meditating on it, it dawned on me how interdependent the phrases of the Mool Mantra really are. For a long time, the Mool Mantra seemed to me a group of adjectives describing the experience of Divinity. But like a seed that breaks open to create roots—what I saw was that the Mool Mantra is not just a description. It defines a process through which we can become aware of the reality of the Divine inside us. Each line describes a state of consciousness; understanding that state becomes a prerequisite to developing an understanding of the state of consciousness described in each succeeding line.

The following prayer is the most well-known prayer of the Sikh faith, not unlike the Lord's Prayer is to people of the Christian faith. This is a very comforting prayer to anyone experiencing a degree of dementia, and all Sikhs relate deeply to its utterance. As we know, the oldest memories we have (especially of childhood) are those which stay with us the longest, even during the most advanced stages of dementia. In fact, we see Alzheimer's victims suddenly come to life when listening to music from their younger days. Some of them are even able to suddenly sing or dance.

In the same way, anyone of the Sikh persuasion will connect with this prayer when a minister will recite it, particularly in the original Gurmukhi language. We are providing the transliteration here for the ease of all providers.

Guru Nanak said (in the opening lines of the Sikh prayer *Japji Sahib*):

Ek Ong Kaar
Saat Naam
Karta Purkh
Nirbhao
Nirvair Akal Moorat
Ajooni
Saibhang
Gurpraasad
Jaap!
Aad Sachh
Jugad Sachh
Hai Bhee Sachh
Nanak Hosee Bhee Sachh

My interpretation/translation of this profound "mantra" of our Divine Essence follows:

One Spirit Beyond moves within the Creation
Coordinating, Consolidating, Continually Creating.
And this Spirit within me is my True Identity.
It Does All and Causes All to be done.
It protects me through all incidents of Time and Space.
It fears nothing and knows nothing of vengeance or anger.
Deathless, it comes into form.
In Itself, It has never been born.

Flowing through the cycles of Birth and Death,
it moves by Its Own Purity and Projection.
This understanding shall come to you as a sweet
blessing, as a gift, through the Guru.
In every moment, continue in its Continual Remembrance.
From the start this Truth was True.
All through Time and Space it is True.
Even now, this Truth is True.
Nanak says, it ever shall be True.

(Excerpted from an article by Ek Ong Kaar Kaur Khalsa Michaud on the Sikh Dharma International website—more at www.sikhdharma.org.)

Chapter 4

CONDUCTING CONGREGATIONAL SERVICES

Dementia-Friendly Congregational Worship

Rev. Karen S. Dumey (Presbyterian Church, USA)

This is the story of how our little church in southeast Missouri, with an average weekly attendance of 30 to 40 people, came to offer a weekly service that includes persons who are affected by Alzheimer's disease and other dementias.

In the spring of 2017, the session (board) of Westminster Presbyterian Church in Cape Girardeau, Missouri, asked the question many small congregations ask: "What can we, a tiny faith community, do to serve God and our community in this time and place?" The immediate response by some was the response commonly heard in aging congregations: "We need to involve more youth, so our congregation will have a future." A micro-congregation with three high school youth is not going to be a magnet for the younger generations. The cost of programming and staffing is too much for a small congregation like Westminster to bear. The leadership talents required are not the God-given talents the members possess. As we debated the merits of this suggestion and the resources required, my question to the session was: "How can our small size be a strength rather than a weakness?"

One of our elders, Susan Smith, answered my question by saying that we should focus on senior citizens rather than youth. She was working with residents at the Missouri Veterans Home in Cape Girardeau and wanted to do more ministry in that direction. At first, Susan's statement did not carry any force as the meeting continued with regular business. But Susan had planted an idea in my head that I could not shake. In following up with Susan, she further refined her initial thought from serving senior citizens to serving persons with Alzheimer's disease and related dementias. This immediately perked my interest, as I have a close family member who has been diagnosed with Alzheimer's disease. Susan and I decided to both go online and see what we could find out about having church services for persons with dementia, and then meet for lunch and compare notes.

I literally Googled "Dementia Worship" and expected to see before me hit after hit on worship styles with outlines of complete liturgies to follow. I had expected the worship aspect of serving those with dementia to be the easy part but was dismayed to find that I was getting few matches for my search. Those I found came primarily from the United Kingdom. I was further disappointed that I did not find a developed liturgy to follow for Sunday worship services. At our follow-up lunch, I discovered that Susan had found the same sites I had.[1]

Undeterred, Susan and I took the next steps in gaining knowledge by attending workshops given by the Greater St. Louis Alzheimer's Association. Here, we learned more about dementia and Alzheimer's disease, as well as the physical and emotional tolls caregivers undergo. Taking our learnings back to our session, we presented the reasons we should become a dementia-friendly congregation, and after discussing the topic and its pros and cons for a few months, we decided to move forward with this as a full ministry. Not only would we offer a dementia-friendly worship experience, but we would expand our pastoral care efforts as well.

Education was the key in bringing forth this new ministry that would affect the entire congregation. First, we learned as a Session, with Susan and me sharing all that we were learning about dementia and Alzheimer's.[2] Then we began teaching the congregation about our new ministry through newsletter articles and after-worship teachings. We taught the members of the congregation how to show hospitality and care for persons with dementia and their caregivers. We discussed the importance of hosting caregiver support groups and dementia evenings out. We learned that being a dementia-friendly congregation included large things like committing ourselves to the pastoral care of individuals not only when people were present in worship, but for the years to come as they were housebound or in a nursing home. We learned that being a dementia-friendly congregation meant we had to overlook the little things, like people walking around the sanctuary, or a person talking when everyone else was quiet. We discussed how to tend to the emotional and spiritual needs of the caregivers as their loved ones

1 The sites initially found and used to develop our dementia-friendly services are: www.dementiamatterspowys.org.uk; www.ageingwellinwales.com

2 *Editors' note*: In the Presbyterian U.S. church, a Session is a governing board usually consisting of the pastor and the other elected (lay) ruling Elders (who are ordained for life).

changed so dramatically before their eyes. Yet, in all our teaching and learning, there was still one problem. How to do worship?

Our research taught us that a 30-minute worship experience worked best. We learnt that music is important, especially the singing of traditional hymns. Repetition or pattern is needed. And that smallness in worship space and in the number of worshipers is important, because too large a space, or too many people, can be overwhelming. (Hurray! Our small size is a strength!) But this left us with a dilemma. While some congregations offer a once-a-month 30-minute Sunday worship experience, we wanted to be a dementia-friendly congregation every Sunday. How could we have a worship experience that lasts 30 minutes for our friends with dementia, and still give our existing congregation the 60-minute worship experience they need and enjoy?

The answer came with something the congregation does each time they gather for worship on a Sunday. During the exchange of the Peace of Christ, almost every member of the congregation pours out of the pews and greets each other in the aisles. This Sunday ritual lasts several minutes. It is an expression of love and welcome found in a bit of chaos. And it is the perfect point in worship for those persons who want or need a 30-minute worship experience to get up out of their seats and exit the sanctuary and without feeling that every person in the congregation is watching them leave. Thus, I rearranged, and rearranged again, the order of our worship experience so that I could get the exchange of peace at that precious 30-minute slot.

Following is the order of worship for our dementia-friendly Sunday services. To create repetition, the order is the same each Sunday, but for three. (The Sunday of the Easter Cantata, the Sunday of the Christmas Cantata, and the Sunday after Easter. On this day we celebrate Upside-Down Sunday and go through the entire liturgy backwards to demonstrate how the Resurrection of Jesus turned our world upside-down.) You will note that I did not include any specific prayers or calls to the order of worship below. If you want to address a specific topic, there are several excellent resources available that you can just insert into this order of worship. For instance, for a caregiver's service, you can go to my denomination's website[3] and get a worship liturgy for such a Sunday.

3 www.pcusa.org

The Prelude
The Choral Introit
Word of Welcome and Announcements
The Opening Prayer
The Call to Worship
Song
First Lesson and Meditation
Sharing Our Lives with One Another
Pastoral Prayer
The Lord's Prayer
Choral Anthem
The Offertory
Doxology
The Prayer of Thanksgiving
Song
Peace of Christ
Call to Confession
Prayer of Confession
Assurance of Pardon
Gloria Patri
A Prayer of Illumination
Scripture Lessons
Sermon
Song
Benediction
The Congregational Response
Postlude

Examining this order of worship, you will see that before the 30-minute point at the Peace of Christ, there are seven places where music occurs. Since music speaks so deeply to most people, including those with dementia/Alzheimer's, it is important to front-load the liturgical music offered. Music is at the core of our service. For us, the prelude is a classical selection played on the organ. Our choir sings the choral introit, which is a short musical selection, about as long in length as singing one verse of a traditional hymn. The song is a traditional hymn sung by the entire congregation. To get a larger selection of traditional hymns to choose from, we use two different hymnals and announce from the pulpit which is the hymnal for the day. By keeping to one hymnal each

Sunday, we lessen some of the confusion that would arise otherwise. Our congregation is trained to glance at those around them and to offer assistance in selecting the proper hymnal, and in finding the correct page. The choral anthem is sung by the choir, and the theme of the selection usually coordinates with the general theme found in the readings and sermon of the day. The offertory is not just a time when the offering is taken up, but another opportunity for music. Our congregation is blessed with talented singers, so their musical offerings are performed here, or a traditional hymn is played on the piano, or another classical piece is played on the organ. Next, we sing the traditional doxology that many people grew up singing: "Praise God, from whom all blessings flow; Praise Him, all creatures here below; Praise Him above, ye heavenly host; Praise Father, Son, and Holy Ghost." And then, another traditional song is sung by the entire congregation.

The music alone takes up much of the 30-minute worship experience. The next question I asked myself was "What are worship essentials?" In our Presbyterian heritage, the reading and preaching of the Word are essential. Yet, I did not have the available time in the first 30 minutes for a sermon. My solution was to include the First Reading and Meditation. Here, I place a scripture reading, followed by a short meditation. I think of the meditation as a children's sermon for adults. In fact, I turn back to children's sermons I have done in the past in order to have a jumping-off point for the meditations I write. The simple illustrations found in children's sermons are perfect to include in a dementia-friendly meditation.

I also considered as essential parts of the worship experience two other things: the occasion to pray together, and the opportunity to support the ministries of the congregation financially through giving. You will note in the order of worship listed above that our prayer time includes saying the Lord's Prayer together and my own pastoral prayer. But this time of prayer begins with sharing our lives with one another. This is a time when anyone in the congregation can share what is going on in their life. It is a time to say, "I had a really good week this past week!" It is a time to share, "I feel myself slipping into depression, and I really need your prayers." While people are urged to share, there is no pressure. Everyone is welcomed just as they are. By offering a time to share our lives with each other, we make stronger the cords of faith and friendship that bind us as a faith community. This one worship element truly fashions who we are as a people—sharing, caring, supportive, prayerful.

As far as including the offering during the first 30 minutes, I think each person should have the chance to give. It is a way to show God our thanksgiving for all of the grace we have received. The generation of people who now have dementia/Alzheimer's is that same generation who were taught by their parents the importance of tithing to the church. They are the same generation who taught their children the importance of tithing. To skip this element of worship would be to skip a part of who this generation is; it would deem them as "less than"; it would not recognize the dignity inherent in each person.

After getting the first 30 minutes in place, the second half of the worship experience was easy to organize because it contains everything else that we typically do during a Sunday service. There is the confession/pardon, the rest of the day's scripture readings, the sermon, and the benediction. There are even five musical components left, including the old familiar Gloria Patri, one more congregational song, a congregational response (this is basically the traveling music that gets the liturgist and me from the chancel to the main doors of the sanctuary before people leave their pews), and the postlude—a final selection of classical music played from the organ.

When it comes to the sacraments of Baptism and Communion, on the Sundays these occur, they are placed after the sermon. Having the placement of Communion in the second half of the worship service does pose a problem, in that for those individuals who leave at the 30-minute mark, they will miss sharing this sacrament with the rest of the congregation. I dislike this breaking of community during such a sacred rite of the church, but the reality is that it is impossible to do everything you want to do in just 30 minutes. For those who are unable to stay for our once-a-month Communion offering, this can be accomplished with home visits where we can further develop our relationships and offer the sacrament in that setting. In this way, no one must go without receiving Communion.

We at Westminster Presbyterian Church in Cape Girardeau are still in the infancy stages of being a dementia-friendly congregation. We are still working to get the word of this ministry out to more people. We are still looking at ways to become more welcoming and supportive. We still look at our facility to see what safety measures may need to be done. But we are grateful. Grateful to have found a ministry where smallness is a strength...grateful that the Holy Spirit is still shaping us and leading us...grateful that the future is no longer a place of fear, but a place of possibility. And we are grateful to all of you who are searching for information, praying for loved ones, learning about dementia/ Alzheimer's, and serving a large population of people so overlooked by our society: our loved ones…our friends…ourselves…with dementia. You and your example give us hope.

African Americans' "Old Timers' Day"

Pastor Bobby Fields, Jr., MDiv (Baptist)

Many churches celebrate the tradition of "Old Timers' Day." This is when the congregation and church officers dress as their grandparents or great-grandparents did for their Sunday worship service. The service is structured to look as much as possible like the services of that day, meaning very little technology beyond the sound system and some instruments is used. The songs all come from that earlier time period and are corporately sung by the congregation. There is usually a fellowship meal afterward and the menu is made up of foods prepared in the manner of that time period, which means none of the food served would find its way onto our modern, healthy menus. While many have abandoned this tradition, it is still alive and well in many African American churches in the South.

There are memories of everyone in their Sunday best sitting in the pews and using the hand-held "church fans," usually from a local funeral home. There are memories of the deacons standing at the front of the church leading the congregation in devotion. They would try and end a song, but someone in the congregation would start singing it again and the congregation would join in with this new song leader. Many remember deacon so-and-so who would get down on a knee and pray too long before the next congregational song began. There was a time for heartfelt testimonies as random members stood and shared how God had blessed them since they were all last together. We are reminded of the altar prayer where it was the preacher's turn to pray too long. We can recall the preacher standing in the pulpit in his robe or his plain black suit, white shirt, and black tie and delivering his sermon in an animated and powerful manner. Many recall the kitchen committee not being in the sanctuary, but still singing and listening to the sermon while they prepared the food. Most can think back to how difficult it was for those in the congregation to focus on the sermon while smelling the delicious food being prepared downstairs or in the fellowship hall next to the main building. Finally, all can remember gathering in the fellowship hall or even outside and eating, conversing, and watching the children play games.

I have found that, in this instance and depending on the size of the congregation, a separate service is not necessary for those with dementia. Why not have a service that is inclusive of all church members—young and old alike, those with cognitive impairments and those who are healthy? This type of service is what our older members grew up in and would be more comfortable in than going into a makeshift room with a few people and having a service that was not as familiar or authentic. This service is beneficial in stimulating the brain to bring out those imbedded memories of the younger years of the person with dementia and getting the general congregation to share the joys of worship. Decorating the walls with photographs or pictures from that time period or just after is also beneficial to memory stimulation, and a way for the congregation to become involved in this spiritual "therapy session" for the day. I have found this service to be enjoyable for all and easily performed. Here is a basic outline of the service along with some suggested songs to utilize:

Old Timers' Day service

Devotional song (deacons)
Prayer (deacon)
Welcome and testimony service
Altar prayer
Choir/congregation songs (2)
Offering (choir sings upbeat song)
Announcements
Choir song
Sermon
Invitation to Christ
Benediction
Fellowship meal

Suggested songs

- Glory, Glory (Since I Laid My Burdens Down)
- Jesus Is on the Main Line

- I Know It Was the Blood
- I'm a Soldier (In the Army of the Lord)
- Trouble in My Way
- What Do You Think About Jesus (He's Alright)
- I Know I've Been Changed
- Somebody Prayed for Me
- Just Another Day that the Lord Has Kept Me
- God Is a Good God (Yes He Is)
- I Feel Like Going On
- This Little Light of Mine

Many people dismiss the warning signs of Alzheimer's, believing that these symptoms, especially short-term memory loss, are a normal part of aging. This is of even greater concern for African Americans, who are *two to three times more likely* to develop late onset Alzheimer's disease than non-Hispanic whites and less likely to have a formal diagnosis of their condition, resulting in less treatment and planning. Alzheimer's affects the entire family, with spouses, sons, daughters, and even grandchildren providing informal, non-professional at-home care for their loved one. This often results in family members having to leave the workforce to provide unpaid care. This is especially true for the African American community where these decisions are driven by economic imperatives and cultural values around taking care of loved ones ourselves.

I offer these observations from the perspective of a family caregiver for my late grandmother, as the former Program Coordinator for Alzheimer's Tennessee, and as an African American pastor. The church still plays a strong role in the lives of those in the African American community, and it is the pastor who often knows more about family members' health than their own primary care physicians.

Walking with Individuals with Dementia and Their Families

An Interfaith Service

Rev. Dr. James W. Ellor (Presbyterian Church, USA)

The celebration of worship in many faith traditions is a time for the members gathered to experience their relationship with fellow believers and their God. Sometimes this reflects faith-specific activities such as prayer or food and fellowship or evangelism, and these may vary considerably from one faith community to another. However, very diverse community churches may also come together to celebrate mutual events such as Lent or Christmas. In each case these events celebrate both common beliefs as well as a desire to share with other groups that may be a bit different but have similar historic understandings of the world.

This article is about our effort to draw the community together to raise awareness, celebrate the life and spirit of persons with dementia, and address the spiritual needs of both the person with dementia and their caregivers. We decided to do this by creating and inviting those interested to attend an *interfaith* worship service. We hoped to support those with dementia and their caregivers, who due to the cognitive, physical, and emotional challenges presented by Alzheimer's are not always able to fully participate in their faith communities. We also wanted to provide a model for diverse congregations to collaborate as a broader community to share efforts and support from a faith perspective.

Many families, as they care for a cognitively impaired relative, become isolated themselves. Often religious traditions offer rituals and rules for how we grieve the death of a relative, but less clear in our various traditions is any prescription for living with and caring for a person with dementia. Not every faith tradition offers specific holy scripture or worship material that speaks directly to memory loss and cognitive impairment. However, with one in every three families being touched by Alzheimer's, every faith group where older adults are present has persons grappling with this disease. In this worship service, a leadership team can draw together as many congregations as possible from the community to reflect a wide variety of faith traditions. The richness of an interfaith service is to suggest that no matter how we understand our own faith tradition, we are all struggling to deal with the same difficulties and needing spiritual support and guidance to sustain us in this most challenging journey. And, people of faith can come together to help each other in a particularly powerful way. The soul does not leave the body when one contracts Alzheimer's disease, and our skills for understanding and ministering to the faith journey of the person must find new forms of expression to be a part of the lives of persons who have a cognitive challenge. An interfaith service can be an important part of this endeavor and would be especially meaningful to offer in November when, as a nation, we recognize both National Alzheimer's Disease Awareness Month and Family Caregivers Month.

This article will discuss both the mechanics of developing such a service as well as some of the lessons learned from our first efforts.

Community worship development

Worship is generally an experience of the sacred as defined by the participant. However, rituals and forms of worship vary from one faith tradition to another. For some, worship is largely prayer, sometimes conducted individually, sometimes in a liturgical context with others. In other traditions, worship includes a variety of music and prayer and other aspects intended to offer spiritual nourishment through that faith tradition. A celebration of interfaith worship can be a joyful time that brings persons of many different faith traditions together in a blended experience that ministers to those with dementia and their caregivers and emphasizes the unity found in families facing the same challenges dementia presents. In this context, every effort to keep any one group from attempting to "proselytize" the others in the group was avoided. Our purpose was not to draw others to any specific faith tradition, but to appreciate the richness that comes from listening to the various ways that other faith traditions are able to experience and make sense of the challenges presented by the various dementias.

Ministering to those with cognitive impairment begins with changing our assumptions about participating in worship. For example, my original model for worship with persons who have dementia was stimulated by a nursing home administrator who did not want dementia patients to come to chapel as they had just put in a new rug and he did not want it to be soiled. As the chaplain, I then designed a program just for the persons on the skilled care unit where the persons with dementia lived, as a carpet should never be the reason anyone is prevented from worship (Ellor, Stettner, and Spath 1987). Clergy tend to assume their parishioners have the capacity to fully understand what is said in the service. This requires both memory and rational thought processes which are slowly lost in the progress of most of the dementias. A person who is unable to remember or to think things through should not be viewed as an inferior person. They are challenged in their cognitive abilities but still have an established sense of who they are, both in their own self-image as well as in the minds of their loved ones. So, we must learn new ways to help them express that personhood and connect with others in meaningful spiritual activities. The celebration of worship is a time for the members gathered to experience their relationship with fellow believers and their God.

Our model for an interfaith service

We drew together leaders from eight different faith traditions to provide a 90-minute celebration and worship experience that was open to the entire Central Texas community. Largely advertised through the local chapter of the Alzheimer's Association as well as participating church newsletters, the sanctuary of the local Presbyterian Church was nearly filled with family members who were caring for loved ones either at home or in long-term care. We encouraged families to bring the impaired senior with them as well. Students from Baylor University's Gerontology Program were available in the back of the church so that if any of the cognitively impaired seniors wanted to get up and take a walk or do something other than sit and listen, they could do so. With the help of the students, they were free to walk around the worship space where sensory stations were set up with things to stop and do or smell or taste. Some of the things they had on hand were fuzzy wall hangings that reflected appropriate symbols, but could be touched, and flowers in solid containers that could be smelled. The students would accompany these individuals, in plain sight of their caregivers, allowing the caregivers to continue to participate in the worship service without having to manage in any way these concerns about their loved ones.

The faith traditions represented were the Presbyterian Church, USA, the United Methodist Church, the Conservative Jewish Community, the Bahá'í Community, three different Baptist traditions, and ELCA Lutheran. One of the local Roman Catholic congregations participated in the planning, but at the last minute their priest was unable to attend. This service was held in Waco, Texas. While there is a great deal of religious diversity in Waco, the two largest traditions are Baptist and Roman Catholic, which suggests that many of the other traditions have only small congregations, and while some faith leaders were interested, they were unable to join our group. Their parishioners were invited to attend the service.

Each pastor involved was invited to prepare a scripture reading, poem, hymn, or other liturgical piece that she/he could present. Each leader was also asked to say a few words of comfort from their faith tradition that might be appreciated by the entire assembly. This allowed each to express various ways of trying to make sense out of dementia and even aging, in the context of their faith traditions. For example, the Rabbi shared a prayer (first in Hebrew and then translated for the assembly) that was focused on how God could bless persons even when the person is not fully aware of what is happening around them. The Bahá'í leader offered a healing prayer from the Baha'u'llah along with an interpretation of what that meant to him and his community. Another expression came from the Methodist pastor as a reflection on Genesis 8.1 on the topic "Does God Remember?" The Lutheran pastor brought a hymn entitled "When Memory Fades" used by permission of Winebrenner Theological Seminary. A Presbyterian pastor reflected on "A Memory of Mother with Alzheimer's Disease." A variety of other familiar hymns, mostly from Christian hymn books, was also shared with the group.

A central part of our service was the "Memory Dedication." Index cards were passed out as people entered the building on which to write the names of their loved ones who they either were caring for now or who had passed away from dementia. These cards were passed forward as an "offering" and then the names read, and the group prayed for by the host pastor. The worship service was opened and closed by the home church pastors.

Lessons learned

The feedback from the participants was overall quite positive. There were expressions of interest as to how other faith traditions thought about the hard questions that individuals were also thinking about and appreciation of new insights from their own faith tradition. The congregation was predominantly Christian; however, Bahá'í, Jewish, and Islamic participants were also in attendance. The one concern raised by some participants was that some of the selections were not always positive or celebrative, as the material was also reflective of some of the very real difficulties of aging and dementia. For instance, not everything in the Christian Bible is positive about the aging experience. But, we had wanted to hold this service in part to share insights and experiences in dealing with these hardships and support each other in our struggles.

When a worship leader selects the elements of their worship service, she or he is in control of all the elements involved and can look over all of the material to understand the gestalt of the entire group of elements of worship. While the organizing committee attempted to do this, it was a challenge to do across so many diverse faith traditions. Based on our experience and this feedback, any new group organizing such a service would be encouraged to be sure that, even with the honest dealing with these adversities, this is primarily a time of celebration and thanksgiving for the lives of the older adults with dementia. It should provide a spiritually elevating experience. Participants need to leave the service feeling encouraged.

Benefits

This event allowed participants an opportunity to gather with members of their geographic community as well as their faith community to worship with the persons living with dementia and to acknowledge the importance of caregivers and families concerned about loved ones with dementia. Reports from the group suggested that this was a unique experience. At the time we developed this service, many congregations were not equipped to accommodate the person with dementia and did not understand how to include them in worship. For many families, the effort to find someone to stay with their loved one so that they can attend worship was a huge challenge. Our service not only encouraged participants to include their loved one with dementia in worship with family and friends, but also offered examples to all the religious leaders present of ways they could manage the manifestations of dementia without disrupting the service.

Finally, each faith tradition offered their own perspective, theological insights, and sacred material or songs that could be appreciated by the others in attendance. The worship bulletin included all the words to each item in the service, allowing participants to re-read and reflect in the future on the various items included. This seemed to be particularly useful to the worship leaders who suggested that they might well borrow some of these ideas in the future.

Community worship in an interfaith context allows neighbors to reach out and care for one another. There are times when caring for a loved one with dementia seems more like hiding them away rather than caring for them and relating to them in a community context. Persons with dementia and their families can feel marginalized or excluded. In this interfaith worship context, these families were able to go to a church, with the impaired senior, celebrate their own faith, and learn about that of their neighbors. In this "dementia-friendly faith community," those living with dementia and their care partners could feel respected, supported, and included in everyday community life.

Reference

Ellor, J.W., Stettner, J., and Spath, H. (1987) 'Ministry with the confused elderly.' *Journal of Religion and Aging* 4, 2, 21–32.

Our interfaith service

Prelude	Local organist
Greeting	Host pastor
Welcome and introduction	Chair of the organizing committee
Expression of the journey	
Experience with a family challenged by a loved one with dementia	Local Methodist pastor
Hebrew reading	Rabbi
Psalm 23	Seminary student
Violin solo	Local choir leader
Bahá'í reading	Bahá'í leader
Romans 5 and a quote from Mother Theresa	Lutheran faith leader
Expression of the loss	
Does God remember? (Genesis 8.1)	Baptist leader
Celebratory prayer	Presbyterian leader
Memory dedication (reading of names on index cards and praying)	Host pastor
Hymn: "When Memory Fades"	Lutheran congregation, sung by congregation
Bahá'í reading on loss	Bahá'í Leader
Brief reflection: "A Memory of Mother with Alzheimer's Disease"	Baptist leader
Celebration of hope for families and community	
Hymns from local hymnal	
Poem: "Response to Ba'al Shem Tov"	Jewish leader
Hymn: "Amazing Grace"	
Benediction	Interfaith committee leader

Chapter 5

PRAYING AND PRAYERS

Prayers of Loving Kindness and Compassion from Buddhism

Olivia Ames Hoblitzelle (Buddhist)

In writing about worship for people with dementia, perhaps the greatest gift we can offer is our presence. We know intuitively when someone has a deeply loving, wise, and compassionate presence. We want to be near them. We trust them, and naturally turn to them for guidance and inspiration. Presence is not something that can be taught; it is the fruit of prayer and meditation, the gift of a life dedicated to contemplation and spiritual practice.

To make the link between the subject of presence and its relevance to dementia, I would like to share a personal story, not only because it is thought-provoking but because it arose from my husband Harrison's lifelong dedication to meditation and the spiritual life. Then, unexpectedly, he was hit with a diagnosis of Alzheimer's. It was when he was in the middle stages of the illness that this simple but profound moment occurred.

By way of background, he had done many meditation retreats, some of which were three months of silence at a time. Eventually he was ordained as a senior teacher, or Dharmacarya, by Thich Nhat Hanh, a much-loved Zen master who teaches worldwide. Harrison taught Buddhist meditation for many years, so when diagnosed with Alzheimer's, he was determined to watch the process of mental diminishment with as much awareness as he could. His practice—and perhaps the luck of how the disease unfolded—surely contributed to his having unusual levels of awareness deep into the illness.

At this particular moment when we were talking, I could see that he was trying very hard to concentrate, gathering his now errant thoughts in a very determined way. Suddenly he looked at me intently and said:

> "This Alzheimer's, it's not to be worried about. It's a different truth."

His words struck me forcefully. Clearly he was lucid, and he had spoken with unusual conviction. I felt he was conveying a very profound message that came from deep spiritual understanding: namely that there is a reality beyond the discursive mind—a sacred realm or ultimate state that is beyond even the ravages of dementia. Prayer or worship of any kind touches us at every level, obviously varying where dementia is present, but this sacred place beyond suffering is also present. And present in everyone.

We may all have heard stories about moments of "terminal lucidity" in dementia patients, when approaching death someone speaks a few words after months or even years of silence, of not having spoken at all. The truth to which Harrison referred is a reminder that we can always reach through the veils of dementia, no matter how advanced, and touch a person with dementia with prayer or loving words even if there is no response.

The power of prayer or meditation will be significantly affected by the *presence* of the person guiding individuals or a group with dementia. With that understanding, I am including two much-loved prayers from the Buddhist tradition, the first from the Theravada (Insight Meditation), the second from Tibetan Buddhism.

One of the most widespread Buddhist meditation or prayer practices is known as *metta*, a word that translates as "loving kindness" or good will, benevolence, or deep caring especially for others. *Metta* is one of the four sublime states known as the Brahmaviharas or *paramis* (perfections) of the Theravada tradition. There are many loving kindness prayers in Buddhism. These prayers are intended to be repeated slowly to let their meaning suffuse one's whole being. The following example is one of many, and the meditator or worship leader is encouraged to find the words that feel most appropriate at the time.

The prayer begins with sending loving kindness to oneself, for one must be able to accept the qualities—or prayerful intentions—that in turn one sends to others. This is a compelling teaching of Buddhism: that prayer/meditation gradually transforms our self-cherishing to compassion for others. All of the lines in the following prayer are traditional, but some of them come from Thich Nhat Hanh, the internationally known Zen master.

May I be peaceful, happy, and light in body and spirit.
May I learn to look upon myself with understanding and love.

May I be free from suffering.
May I have deepest well-being.
May I be able to recognize and touch the seeds of joy and happiness in myself.
May I have ease of heart and deep contentment.
May I be able to live with awareness, equanimity, and freedom.

May all beings be peaceful, happy, and light in body and spirit.
May all beings learn to look upon themselves with understanding and love.
May all beings be free from suffering.
May all beings have deepest well-being.
May all beings be able to recognize and touch the seeds of joy and happiness in themselves.
May all beings have ease of heart and deep contentment.
May all beings be able to live with awareness, equanimity, and freedom.

Sometimes for people with dementia, we may need a simpler form of prayer, especially if you're with someone one-to-one. The following prayerful words are very simple, calming, and beautiful. One explains to the person with dementia that we will be quiet together, and all they have to do is listen.

Then as the guide, you say the phrases very slowly, allowing a couple of breaths or more between each phrase. If you can coordinate the phrases with their in breath and out breath, that is even more helpful.

> "Clear mind...peaceful heart. Clear mind...peaceful heart. Clear mind... peaceful heart."

If they are agitated, you might consider using the words "Quiet mind... peaceful heart."

The quiet repetition can be very calming, sometimes easing the person into sleep. Realistically, however, we all know that sometimes an agitated person may have a hard time following any form of prayer.

The following prayer comes from the Tibetan tradition and has a somewhat different intent. It is called the Dalai Lama's Bodhicitta Prayer (the word *bodhicitta* means "awakened heart/mind"), because it has its origins many centuries ago in his particular lineage, and he encourages those who attend his teachings to include this prayer as part of their practice.

To briefly explain words that may be unfamiliar: to take refuge in the Buddha is to acknowledge our connection not only to the historical Buddha but to all the wise ones—to wisdom itself, to compassion, loving kindness, and all the inspiring qualities that one such as the Buddha embodies. The second refuge is the *dharma*, a Sanskrit word for the truth or the way to the truth, which would include the teachings, the practices, devotion—all the elements of the spiritual path. And the third refuge is the *sangha*, or community—everyone from our fellow seekers to the wise ones of all times, from all traditions.

This prayer would have familiar elements for all Buddhists whatever their particular tradition. The prayer carries the strong intention that we might awaken and ultimately become enlightened for the sake of all beings, dedicating our lives to alleviating suffering wherever it appears.

DALAI LAMA'S BODHICITTA PRAYER

With a wish to free all beings,
We always go for refuge
To the Buddha, Dharma, and Sangha
Until we reach full enlightenment.

Inspired by wisdom and compassion,
Today, in the Buddha's presence,
We generate the mind of full awakening
For the benefit of all beings.

As long as space remains,
As long as sentient beings remain,
Until then may we too remain
And dispel the miseries of the world.

In sharing these Buddhist prayers, may they inspire all those who hear them. May they deepen in compassion, wisdom, and loving kindness.

The Lord Be With You!

Rev. Dr. Cynthia Huling Hummel (Presbyterian Church, USA)

Try as it might, Alzheimer's couldn't touch my mom's deep faith and love of the church. She simply loved going to Mass. She remembered the holy water and how to bless herself in the name of the Father, Son, and Holy Spirit. Mom remembered to take a bulletin and to genuflect before the cross before she went into the pew. She remembered all the responses in the Mass and said them with confidence with a hint of theatrics as she nodded to others to make sure that we knew that she knew the words! Mom knew when to stand and when to sit. She knelt as the priest held the host high. As the chimes rang, Mom beat her fist against her breast. She walked forward to receive communion knowing that someone would guide her back to the pew. Mom remembered all the words to "Holy, Holy, Holy," "Eagle's Wings," and "Be Not Afraid," and she sang them with gusto. She would reach for the offering envelope that my dad had slipped into her purse before we left the house and proudly put it in the basket that the ushers passed. Mom loved the passing of the peace. She would admire babies, smile at everyone, and shake hands, saying, "The peace of Christ be with you," and it was, thanks to Mom and her contagious faith.

On the night before she died, I kissed her goodbye and tucked her in. The TV in her room was playing one commercial after another, so I decided to try and find something more soothing for her to listen to. As I flipped the channels of the remote, I couldn't believe it: a Latin Mass. Truly a gift from God! And from somewhere far away, Mom smiled at the familiar words from her childhood, "Dominus, vobiscum," "The Lord Be With You," a blessing and promise: God's lullaby—rocking her to sleep and tenderly calling her home.

Prayer for a Fellow Soldier

Rev. Bob Inkenbrandt (Nondenominational Christian)

Beloved Father in heaven,
Jesus, my King and glorious Savior,
Holy Spirit, great and mighty Counselor and Comforter;
Look upon this servant with kindness and gentle mercies.
Grant this heart, mind, and body rest from the weariness of battle.
May Your great comfort and care restore and renew.
May Your peace wash over this soul, cleansing and healing like the forgiving blood shed by You on the cross, Lord Jesus.
Give strength where strength is needed, hope that never dies, and love that forever welcomes.
In the name of the Father, Son, and Holy Spirit I pray.

Pray Psalm 55.16–18 (*New International Version*)

16
As for me, I call to God,
and the Lord saves me.

17
Evening, morning, and noon
I cry out in distress,
and he hears my voice.

18
He rescues me unharmed
from the battle waged against me,
even though many oppose me.
Amen.

Veterans face an increased risk for dementia stemming from post-traumatic stress disorder (PTSD), depression, traumatic brain injury (TBI), successive concussion syndrome, and blast-induced neurotrauma (BINT). Some may experience what we call *moral injury* and may have unresolved grief and guilt, anger, and alienation issues that still need addressing. Through prayer we can offer understanding, comfort, support, forgiveness, and peace.

A Prayer for Forgotten Souls

Chaplain Maria Khani (Muslim)

In a world full of chaos, we sometimes come across loved ones who find themselves unknowingly trapped beneath a darkness, an ailment not just of the body, but of the mind. They are trapped beneath the darkness we today call dementia.

Throughout my years of chaplaincy, working with inmates, I have encountered those who were incarcerated physically and those who were incarcerated both physically and mentally. The most challenging groups I have faced, however, are those who have been incarcerated physically, mentally, and spiritually.

One of my favorite stories in the Quran is that of Moses and the burning bush. Moses told his family that he would bring them a brand from the fire he sees, to make them feel warm and secure. When he arrived, he was surprised that there was no fire, but a light, and that that light was the presence of his Lord.

Darkness is only the absence of light!

Those who struggle with dementia and those who are incarcerated live in a dark world. They are isolated from their loved ones and fear overwhelms them, making it even more difficult to cope with their surroundings. Regardless of what they say, or even don't say, they need someone like Moses who can bring them some light to brighten their journey and make them feel safe and secure.

The power of prayer may not come in the changing of destiny, even though miracles do happen, but prayer's power is evident in showing love, hope, and support to those who receive them.

A prayer is a state of humility in the presence of the Lord. It is a complete trust in the Lord, the All Mighty, the Loving and the Powerful One, Who can change all circumstances. It is a state of accepting reality that is under no one's control except the Lord's.

A prayer is an acknowledgment of God's blessings, and it is indeed powerful enough to reach souls, minds, and hearts in moments where nothing else can touch them.

I share my prayer with those afflicted by the darkness, whose souls are calling for the Light.

I share it with their families and their caregivers and with those whom God knows are in need of prayers.

Quran–40.60. "And your Lord said: Call Me and I will answer your prayer."

Gracious Lord:
* *You are the Creator of Heaven and Earth and everything in between*
* *You are the Creator of the mountains, the oceans, and every living thing*
* *You are the Loving God and the Truth*
* *You are the Sufficient One and everything depends on You*

Lord of the Universe:
* *You bring the day after the night*
* *You calm the ocean after the storm*
* *You bring the sun after the rain*
* *Your Mercy and Knowledge encompasses all things and nothing can encompass You*

Loving God:
* *You are the First and You are the Last*
* *You created us from naught and we are grateful*
* *You gave us life and we praise You*
* *You are in charge and we trust You*

Lord All Mighty:
* *You gave us knowledge when we were ignorant*
* *You gave us strength when we were weak*
* *You gave us from Your Bounty before we even asked*
* *You are the Provider and we are thankful*

Powerful God:
* *You see our hearts and purify them*
* *If we are alive it is through Your Grace*
* *If we were dead it is our Destiny*
* *If we are sick it is Your Will*

Dear God, the Lord of Mankind:
* *How can we depend on anyone when the Universe depends on You?*
* *How can we trust anyone before we trust You?*
* *How can we ask anyone before we ask You?*

God All Knowing:
* *You alone are worthy of worship and from You alone we seek help*
* *You know what we want and we may not know what is best*
* *You answer our prayers when we raise our hands*
* *Help us to call Your name not only when we are in need*

God, the Healer:
* *You are able to do all things*
* *You make the impossible possible*
* *You are the Healer and we seek Your Mercy*
* *Heal our hearts, souls, minds, and bodies*

Lord, Who listens to our prayers:
* *If we lose hope in things, never let us lose hope in You*
* *If we are sick and impatient, let us be patient through You*
* *If we are too weak to ask, keep us under Your Eyes*
* *If we are healed by Your Grace, let us always be grateful*

God, You are the Protector:
* *We pray for all who are patients—souls and bodies, hearts and minds*
* *Lighten their burden and ease their journey*
* *We pray for their families to continue supporting their loved ones*
* *We pray for the caregivers, for their love and compassion and strength in their mission*
* *We pray for the souls who left us, to be granted Forgiveness and Mercy*
* *We pray for all those who are in need of help in the World*
* *We seek refuge in You from the evil*
* *We pray for all and for love and peace*
* *We pray not to be forgotten*

In Your Holy Name,

Amen

The Intimate Touch of Meditative Prayer

Carlen Maddux (Presbyterian Church, USA)

Three weeks after turning 50, my wife Martha was diagnosed with early onset alzheimer's.[1] The date was September 23rd, 1997. Anyone familiar with this disease will understand when I say, "Our life wasn't turned upside down. It imploded before us."

But our story is not about the fallout from this insidious disease, which extended over 17 years. Rather, it's the story of a path emerging "during our darkest hours, a path that we neither planned nor foresaw."

After the doctor handed down his verdict, we rushed home having no idea what to do. Yet Martha did know one thing: She did *not* want to tell anyone—not our children, not her parents, not our closest friends. There was one person, however, she was willing to share with—a retired Presbyterian minister named Rev. Lacy Harwell. She and Lacy were friends before we got together; he married us and baptized two of our children; and we remained close throughout our 25 years of marriage.

After sharing and crying with Lacy, followed by a long silence, he told us about his friend and confidante, Sister Elaine Prevallet. "A number of my friends faced with a serious crisis have gone to visit Elaine. I've never met another person with her gift of discernment. I don't know where your visit might lead, but it would be worth your time and effort."

And so three weeks after being hit with the news of alzheimer's, we drove out of St. Petersburg, Florida, to visit Sr. Elaine at the Sisters of Loretto community in Kentucky, an hour south of Louisville. This is not the place to get into all that we discussed during our week's visit, but as we left she told us two things: "Your main calling at this time is to trust that you belong to God and not to yourselves. And to deepen your love for God and between yourselves."

---

1 In my book *A Path Revealed* (2016) I chose not to capitalize the disease known as alzheimer's. With all due respect to Dr. Alois Alzheimer, who identified this dementia a century ago, I felt that its name doesn't deserve the respect conferred by its capitalization. And so I won't capitalize it here either.

And the other thing that Sr. Elaine suggested: that we check into the ancient practice of meditation. Yet she offered no more insight than that. Though I was curious about meditation, or contemplative prayer, I was also skeptical.

After returning home, we shared with Lacy the highlights of our visit. I then asked him what he knew about meditation. "Catholics have a rich heritage of this," he said. "Protestants don't." Lacy pointed us to a Benedictine monk named Fr. John Main. "He's the best I've found. He's really good at making meditation understandable to the average person."

I went online and found a book of John Main's, *Word into Silence* (2016), and a set of tapes, *In the Beginning* (1988).

And Martha and I began to meditate, a practice we continued off-and-on throughout our 17-year odyssey. We sat side-by-side on our couch, holding hands as I whispered aloud the word we had chosen to say. We meditated for 15–20 minutes in the morning and in the evening as best we could.

Nothing happened immediately other than I became acutely aware of all the distractions reverberating in my mind. Over time, though, my anxiety diminished. And I also sensed a gathering calm within Martha. She was more relaxed as her confidence showed signs of returning.

But something even more profound emerged, something I'd not anticipated. I sensed an intimacy growing between us that we'd not experienced in our 25 years of marriage. It was a warm, unspoken bond arising from deep within.

Let's step back for a moment so I might explain how we moved into this ancient practice:

- First, meditation is a form of prayer in which you seek to listen for God's quiet voice rather than informing God of your requests and needs. Not that making requests is wrong, but for me that's more like a first step into the fullness of prayer.

- We had no mentor who could direct us. If you do, draw fully on him or her. Lacy Harwell could have been our mentor but he was out of town more often than in. Nonetheless, John Main's (2016) book, *Word into Silence*, and tapes (now CDs), *In the Beginning* (1988), were excellent guides. Having both was vital to my understanding of how to proceed. They still are.

- It's important to find an approach that you're comfortable with. Early on I was using both John Main's guides and Thomas Keating's (1997) book on centering prayer, *Open Mind, Open Heart*. These are two different, effective approaches. I was getting confused as to which was the "right" way. After awhile, I realized that we just needed to pick one of the paths. They both lead to the same object—a return to God's wholeness.

- You should find a quiet place to sit straight and still—comfortably, not rigidly.

- John Main says to meditate twice a day, 20–30 minutes in the morning and 20–30 minutes in the evening. It's also beneficial to meditate occasionally with others. Our church has a group that meets once every two weeks.

- If you're like me, it was difficult at first to meditate for 20 minutes. There was too much flak flying around in my mind. If so, you might start at five minutes and build up to 20–30 minutes. Once you have, meditate your prescribed time no matter what. If you find the going slow and difficult, stick to your prescribed time. If your effort is grace-filled and easy, stick to your prescribed time and no more.

- John Main suggests using the Aramaic word *Maranatha*, which essentially means "Come, Lord." (It's one of the last phrases in the book of Revelation, chapter 22.20 specifically.) Repeat your word, or mantra, slowly in your mind, as in *mah-rah-nah-thah*. (I obviously whispered our word aloud so Martha could follow along.) You may wish to tie the word to your breathing: breathe in—*mah-rah*; breathe out—*nah-thah*.

- Continue to repeat *mah-rah-nah-thah* slowly in your mind throughout your allotted time, paying attention to the *sound* of your word rather than its meaning.

- As you meditate, you will get distracted and find yourself thinking of something else. Don't worry; just return to your word by repeating it slowly in your mind.

- John Main emphasizes three qualities necessary to proceed with meditation: *persistence*, *patience*, *attentiveness*. There's nothing magical or dramatic about meditation. "It's extraordinary in its ordinariness." He makes clear that no matter how long we've practiced meditation, we're always beginners.

- Finally, I leave this ancient Eastern Orthodox saying with you, which Sr. Elaine Prevallet shared with us: *Fold the wings of your mind. Place your mind in your heart. Come into the presence of God.*

If you're a member of the clergy and are unfamiliar with this form of prayer, but interested, what can you do to proceed? A few thoughts come to mind:

- It doesn't matter whether you're an "expert" or not. In fact, it might be better if you're not.
- Form a meditation group with you or another as the leader. Invite individuals and couples with a serious crisis, whether it's alzheimer's or something else. Also invite those not dealing with a serious crisis (they'll probably have one sooner or later).
- In our church's group, we listen to a John Main homily for 15–20 minutes and meditate for 20 minutes. Early on we started with 10 minutes. Afterwards, you may have a question/discussion time, or not. Our group is in and out within an hour, entering quietly and leaving quietly.
- If a couple in the group is struggling with an issue like dementia, it's probably a good idea for them to hold hands as they meditate. That non-verbal touch is so important.
- If an individual with dementia is still capable of attending such a group, you might invite their closest friend to attend and share this experience with them.
- When you visit someone with dementia in a nursing home, don't think you need to fill your visit with conversation. Often sitting nearby, praying or meditating silently, will be sufficient. Other helpful suggestions are referenced throughout this book.
- More information about meditation can be found on the World Community for Christian Meditation (WCCM) website.[2] This

---

2 www.wccm.org

organization grew out of John Main's teachings and is led by his protégé, Fr. Laurence Freeman.

As we know, dementia and alzheimer's mess with a person's verbal skills and mental processes. And after enough frustration, dementia messes with the emotions of both the victim and the caregiver. Martha was high energy and verbal, but as her skills declined, we were forced to find non-verbal activities to help bring her out of her shell. Dancing and singing were key. Also vital was the unfolding interest in art, a talent she'd never exhibited before.

What role do I now see that meditation played through the volatile, early years of our odyssey? In hindsight, I believe that it was a foundational practice that helped encourage the re-emergence of Martha's confidence. She was able to connect again with those around her, but at a different level from which we'd been used to.

After practicing meditation for two decades, I know that it helps me on several fronts. The most important, I feel, is that it continues to move me from a judgmental, performance-based mindset to one that's more relational and loving.

Let's go back to the year 2010. More than a decade after her diagnosis, Martha was living in the Menorah Manor nursing home. By now she could not talk, she could not walk, and she couldn't feed herself. When I visited, Martha frequently was curled up in her bed or chair, in a fetal position. As I approached, I'd say, "Hi Martha, this is Carlen." Sometimes she'd recognize me, often not.

I would sit beside her and slip my hand into hers, trying to let her know she was not alone. And then I would slip into a quiet meditation, whispering the word we'd shared all these years. More often than not Martha relaxed, unfolding her body. A calming presence frequently arose, like a quiet song in the distance, caressing Martha as it caressed me. Her agitation ceased; my mind's chatter halted; all was still.

As I reflected on such moments, this quiet "presence" seemed to have everything to do with God's commitment to Martha and her well-being. And to our children and their families, as well as to me.

And I often wondered, "Is this the healing presence of Christ Jesus?"

References

Keating, T. (1997) *Open Mind, Open Heart: The Contemplative Dimension of the Gospel*. New York: Continuum.

Maddux, C. (2016) *A Path Revealed: How Hope, Love and Joy Found Us Deep in a Maze Called Alzheimer's*. Orleans, MA: Paraclete Press.

Main, J. (1988) *In the Beginning*. 6 tapes, 12 homilies. Montreal: The Benedictine Priory.

Main, J. (2016) *Word into Silence: A Manual for Christian Meditation*. Norwich: Canterbury Press.

Prayer in a Jewish Long-Term Care Facility

Rabbi Dr. James R. Michaels (Jewish)

I'll begin this article by telling a story about the desire to pray of a woman with dementia. She had been admitted to our skilled nursing facility for rehabilitation after a fall. She had lived for several years in a non-denominational care setting, but her daughter thought she would do better in a facility with a Jewish religious and cultural ambience. I'll call her "Goldie," although it's not her real name.[3] Goldie had never been one to attend religious services, although her parents had been Orthodox Jews. Girls were typically not given a religious education, and she continued this pattern throughout her adult life.

Goldie had, however, sent her daughter to Hebrew School, so she was attuned to Jewish prayer and felt comfortable in synagogue. Goldie's husband had died a few months before, and her daughter was observing the year of mourning for her father; she wanted to attend our daily religious services to say the mourner's Kaddish. She brought Goldie with her; she prayed while Goldie sat in her wheelchair.

Goldie was discharged from rehab and moved to one of our long-term care units. Her daughter told me, "You might want to ask her if she wants to attend services, but I doubt that she'll want to go." The next day, I went to her room and asked if she wanted to join us for the morning service. She was delighted to be asked. I brought her to the synagogue, and put her wheelchair in an open space. She sat without a prayer book, listening to the words, chants, and songs. She seemed to like it.

The next day, I asked if she wanted to join us again. To my surprise, she remembered she had done so the day before, and said she would love to come. "I'm a good Jewish girl," she said. "I should be in synagogue." I brought her again, to her continued enjoyment. The following day, I asked her again, and she gave the same response, but this time in Yiddish. She had an even bigger smile. This began a pattern of Goldie's attending

3 All residents in this article will be identified by pseudonyms.

our religious services twice each day. In her nineties, having never gone regularly to synagogue, she now had found a new focus for every day.

What was it that Goldie found so attractive and enticing? It could have been the words and melodies of the prayers. Or perhaps it was the regularity of going twice each day; the nostalgia for the sounds and feelings of her youth; or simply a reinforcement for her Jewish identity. Any of these is possible. And it demonstrates that Jewish prayer can be very important for people with dementia. (I'll return to Goldie's story later.)

The nature of Jewish prayer

A Jewish service is text-driven. When someone goes into a synagogue for a religious service, he/she is given a Siddur (prayer book) and directed to turn to the page where the service will begin. The entire service—prayers, hymns, Scripture reading—is included in the Siddur. With occasional exceptions, Jews in synagogue won't need to look at any other text.

Jews traditionally pray three times each day—morning, afternoon, and evening—although the latter two services are usually said one after the other. There is a standard format for each service, always found in the Siddur. This format consists of traditional Hebrew prayers. Jews who have been raised in a religious environment will usually be familiar with at least some of the prayers, especially those which are sung or chanted aloud.

Jewish prayers are "davened." That is, the words are usually chanted, sometimes individually and often in unison. The melodies of these chants are well known. Children learn them when they are very young and often memorize them. The same is true with certain essential prayers, such as the Sh'ma ("Hear, Israel, the Lord is our God; the Lord is one"). It's recited twice each day, in a melody so ingrained that even people with advanced dementia will chant it aloud with the congregation. And it's all found in the Siddur.

Familiarity with these prayers presents an opportunity for those who lead services for people with dementia. That is, since many of the prayers and melodies are ingrained in patients' long-term memories, singing or reading them aloud will allow them to access deep-set memories. Even if a patient hasn't been active in religious activities for a long time, he/she will often respond favorably to the service's words and melodies.

The challenge to those who serve elderly people with dementia is how to provide a Siddur which suits their physical and mental needs. The print must be large; the book should be light enough for frail fingers, yet sturdy enough to withstand torn pages; the format of the service should be fast-paced, yet not too subtle for people to lose interest. In addition, in a senior care residence, there's usually only one service which must cater to people from the various branches of Judaism (Orthodox, Conservative, Reconstructionist, and Reform).

Creating specialized prayer books

The Charles E. Smith Life Communities serves the people of Washington D.C., including suburban Maryland and Northern Virginia. There are six buildings providing 1100 residents with skilled nursing, independent living, assisted living, and memory care. I have served as Director of Pastoral Care for the facility since 2003. When I began my tenure, every building used standard-printed Siddurim for their services. Over the years, we have created specialized volumes to meet the needs of the residents in each building. The impetus to do this was, as mentioned above, because the needs of the residents differed from setting to setting.

Over the years, we've created six different volumes of prayer. At first, I would simply make photocopies of pages in published prayer books, cut the material I wanted to use, and then paste them into the desired format. More recently, I've used available Hebrew software programs from Davka and Nissus. For English translations, I've used English word processing programs.[4] The aim has been to create books which will satisfy the needs of the residents in our various buildings:

- Residents in independent living and assisted living requested services which maintained a traditional feel, including well-known prayers and melodies, but not lasting as long as traditional services.
- Residents in our skilled nursing facility needed a truncated service which nonetheless contained all or most of the elements of traditional prayer services.

4 For more details, see "Technology to Enhance Religious Life" (Chapter 15) in Michaels and Kozberg (2011).

- The residents in our memory care building don't use books, but still enjoy hearing the sounds and words of traditional prayers.[5]

With the exception of the residents in memory care, we discussed the project of creating new prayer books with the residents who would use them. They contributed some very good suggestions. These included English readings, transliterations of Hebrew into English characters—especially for passages which would be sung aloud—and a book which would be light in weight but still large enough to accommodate large print.

In the process of composing and editing various Siddurim, I discovered the important points below.

Create a volume which looks professional and pleasing

The residents take pride in what they're using for prayer services. They don't want photocopied pages which are stapled together. Our volumes are all printed professionally, using glossy covers and spiral bindings.

Hebrew and English page orientations

Most residents want a book which opens from the right; they view it as a Hebrew book, even though it contains English translations. I've noticed, however, that some residents get confused by this format. The leader will announce a page change, and they'll turn the page from left to right, as would be done in an English book. They are then bewildered and may blurt out "I don't have that page!" or "What's the matter with this book?" To deal with this, I ordered a few books printed from left to right, as an English volume. (To distinguish them from the Hebrew-oriented books, I've used a different color plastic spiral binding.) This has been effective and useful for a few residents.

Allocate sufficient time for the project

The work of creating a new book, especially one which is professionally produced, can take a long time. I started creating each book a year before

5 See "Memory Care and Shabbat" by Andrea (Yonina) Foster in this book.

I planned to begin using it. This allowed me the opportunity to create, compile, edit, and proofread the text before sending it to the printer.

Make a "beta"

I found it was best to test the volumes in real-time situations over a period of several months. This allowed the opportunity for feedback from residents about what they liked, and what needed improvement. In addition, no matter how much I tried to catch typos and formatting errors, inevitably some would not be found. Creating a "beta" volume removed pressure because we could always include corrections on the second, final edition.

Creating a meaningful prayer environment

The process of producing new prayer books has resulted in a very special environment within the larger care-giving facility. Applying clinical principles to the task of leading daily services has resulted in many benefits for our residents who attend.

Creating a sacred space

The nature of any health care facility is going to be busy and perhaps noisy. Our religious services, on the other hand, are relaxed and conducive to meditation. They even attract some residents who may never have participated in a praying community. They welcome the opportunity to sit and interact with residents from other residential units. One man told me, "I come because I like the quiet." And since most people attend every day, they get to know each other, if only to nod in recognition.

Recognition of different religious needs

While some residents have been attending traditional services for their entire lives, others may have belonged to Reform or Reconstructionist congregations. By including English readings in every service, and working within prescribed limits so the service isn't overly long, we've created a space where liberal Jews are comfortable and feel respected.

Including members of the greater community

Our facility has offered religious services for most of its 107-year history. It is well known that our services are open to the community; almost every day, someone will come in and join us. Many attend because they are saying Kaddish,[6] and others come to pray with their parents or other relatives. Their presence conveys an important message to our residents: they haven't been left behind. In fact, since they provide the required quorum of ten people, the residents understand that they are doing something useful.

Promoting intergenerational interaction

Every summer, many high school students volunteer in our skilled nursing buildings. Their primary motivation is to complete 60 hours of community service, required for graduation. Many of these students continue to volunteer after the minimum requirement is fulfilled. They do so because they become familiar with the residents, especially those who attend services. They sit next to the residents and assist them with turning pages, or chanting parts of the service. Some continue during the school year, picking a specific day each week to come and interact with the residents. (I admit to a special bias on this matter, since my own grandchildren come to our services whenever they visit us. One even chose to have her Bat Mitzvah ceremony in our synagogue.)

Mixing old and new melodies

Since our clientele all suffer some memory loss, we have found it best to chant or sing the prayers using traditional melodies. We have, on occasion, introduced newer melodies. We do this by including the words in transliteration (i.e. English characters) in the prayer books. We also sing these melodies every day, so they become ingrained in residents' long-term memory. By doing this, we have introduced some variety in the service while maintaining a traditional format.

---

6 Jews who have recently lost a relative traditionally say the Kaddish, a mourner's prayer, in the aftermath of their relative's death. It is recited for a year after a parent dies, and for a month for other near relatives. Afterward, they will say Kaddish on the anniversary of the death. Since it is recited in a communal setting, mourners will seek out a service where the required quorum of ten will be found.

Dementia details

So, all these elements are in place, and our various facilities are ready to host daily, Sabbath, and holiday services. Volunteers are assigned to escort residents to the service, since most are sitting in wheelchairs. They begin at least 30 minutes in advance, and the synagogue or meeting hall begins to fill up. The rabbi or lay person assigned to lead the service takes his/her place at the front of the room. What are some of the things the leader must do or avoid?

Don't say, "Please rise"

Ministers, priests, and rabbis are taught to give directions about the proper position for a song or prayer. (Ideally, lay persons should be so familiar with the service that they wouldn't need this prompt, but that's too much to hope for.) Having spent a career giving these directions, it's hard to break the habit. But people in wheelchairs, especially those with dementia, may take that instruction literally and try to stand. That, in turn, could lead to more serious problems, such as falling.

As mentioned above, members of the community often come to attend services with residents. When they don't get directions to stand, they look at each other, and to the leader, with quizzical looks. If possible, before the service begins, we explain they won't be hearing what they expect, and they should understand we're not trying to confuse them; instead, we're interested in patients' safety.

Speak up

I've noticed that clergy of all denominations tend to speak softly when they speak to people individually while they're in a service. (Is there a theological point to this? It has never been explained to me.) But older people, especially those with dementia, tend to be hard of hearing. I tell our prayer leaders not to use "indoor voices" when they're in front of the residents, or even next to them. Loud voices are altogether appropriate in these settings.

Familiar gestures

In Jewish services there are times when the leader will carry the Torah scroll around the congregation. Jews are taught from a very young age that when a Torah is brought near, they should show reverence and love by kissing it. This is usually done by reaching out one's hand, touching the scroll, and then kissing the hand; those wearing a *tallit* (prayer shawl) will use it to touch the scroll, and then kiss the fringes on the end. This practice is so ingrained that even deeply demented people will do it. In fact, it may be a highlight of the service. Some who have limited mobility with their arms or hands may want to kiss the scroll directly with their mouths; they should be allowed to do it.

Taking an "aliya"

When the Torah is read in the synagogue, lay people are invited to come and recite the appropriate blessing. The blessing is called an "aliya," which means "going up." (This is because, in synagogues, the Torah is read on a raised platform; hence one "goes up" to recite the blessing.) Most men were taught this blessing as they prepare for their Bar Mitzvah ceremonies.[7] Since the blessing is so well imbedded in residents' memories, it's important to include opportunities for people to take the aliya, even if they can't read or remember any other prayers.

Carrying and lifting the Torah scroll

In 2006, a generous donor endowed a project where a Torah scroll was written especially for us. Working with a scribe, we specified that the scroll should be small, light in weight, and easy to lift. When it was complete, we were able to allow some residents to carry the scroll during the service. Even while sitting in a wheelchair, they can easily hold the scroll while others reach out to touch or kiss it. Some even have sufficient upper body strength to lift it. Residents who do this always have a look of delight, mirrored by the smiles on the faces of other residents as well as their family and friends.

7 Today, most girls are given the same education; since many older women didn't have a Bat Mitzvah ceremony as girls, they may have one as an adult. Some women in our facility have had the ceremony in their 80s or 90s.

Spirituality in elder care settings

Ultimately, the goal of all this has been to create an environment which our residents will find conducive to their need and desire to pray. Here are some stories which have taken place in our various services.

I'll begin, again, with Goldie. Once she started coming to services, she began to recall the experiences of her childhood in Baltimore. She recalled that her parents didn't send her to learn Hebrew, although her younger brother learned it. She started to complain that she couldn't read the Hebrew in the prayer book; she also was confused by the Hebrew orientation of the prayer book. Since we had the English-oriented book for her, she was much more at ease when we announced a page change. And even though she couldn't read the Hebrew, she was very proud that she could turn each page at the designated time. She continues to come to services twice each day. And she says she's hoping her brother (now deceased) will come and teach her to read the Hebrew.

"Sarah" was a woman with a relatively high cognition level. Although she had not been very active in her synagogue, she became friendly with several residents who attended services every day. They encouraged her to start doing so too, and she quickly took an interest in the prayers, the Torah reading, and the atmosphere of the service. She saw other men and women taking aliyas, and asked if she could do so too. We gave her a copy of the Hebrew blessings, written out in transliterated English. It was not a challenge for her to do so.

After a few months, I met Sarah's daughter for the first time. She hadn't known that her mother was attending services every day, so I invited her to join us. We brought Sarah to the Torah scroll, where she proudly read the blessing while her daughter stood next to her. She had tears in her eyes as she saw that her mother was actually growing and learning with us.

"Abe" was a retired rabbi with advanced Alzheimer's. In his prime, Abe was well respected for his skills in a congregation in Manhattan. He was also very active in interfaith work, earning recognition from the Anti-Defamation League and also an honorary degree from a Catholic university. I had known him when I was a young rabbi in New York City, and was surprised when he was admitted into a dementia unit in our facility. (As with so many of our residents, he and his wife had moved to the DC area to be near their daughter.) Despite his dementia, Abe could still use a walker and was often escorted to our Sabbath service by his wife, who lived in one of our independent living buildings.

One Saturday morning, Abe was sitting in the front row while I was leading the service. He suddenly stood up and walked to the lectern and turned to face the other residents in the congregation. I asked if he wanted to lead, and he said yes. He then took the prayer book and read every prayer in Hebrew. He even knew when to turn to the Ark (where the Torah scrolls are kept) and bowed at the appropriate times. After about 20 minutes, he seemed to be tiring. I asked if he wanted to return to his seat and he agreed. Worrying that the other residents might have resented having him lead, I asked how they felt about it. Without hesitation, one woman shouted out, "That hit the spot!"

Another man, "Sol," was brought to our skilled nursing building after living for many years in Florida. He had been religious all his life, and his daughter requested that we bring him to services every day and assist him to wear tefillin.[8] Various members of our team of "religious assistants" brought him to the synagogue and put them on his arm and forehead. We were never sure if he could read the prayers from the prayer book, but he seemed to be at ease throughout the service.

One summer, Sol was befriended by one of our CPE interns, a student studying for the ministry at Virginia Theological Seminary in Alexandria, VA. This young man enjoyed sitting next to Sol every morning during services; he was particularly interested in how he would wear the phylacteries. I eventually asked him if he would like to learn how to assist Sol. When he agreed, I showed him a book with explicit instructions. He then helped Sol for the next five weeks. Toward the end of his training, I asked the student how he would use this experience in the future. He responded, "God only knows"; he knew that one day this lesson would be important in his ministry. (Sol died two days after the intern completed his internship.)

8 Known in English as "phylacteries," these are leather boxes which contain four passages from the Torah instructing Jews to "bind them as a sign upon your hand, and they shall be a frontlet between your eyes." Hand written on parchment, these passages are inserted in the boxes, which are worn on the upper arm and upper forehead, affixed by leather straps. Traditionally worn by men, today some women are also performing this commandment.

"Rivka" was a 98-year-old woman. Although confined to a wheelchair, she would ambulate herself into our Sabbath services every Saturday morning. Legally blind, she would sit at the rear of the room and listen to the sounds and words of the service. One Saturday, I was surprised when she left her usual spot and came toward the front of the room. She said aloud, "Please ask God to forgive me. I couldn't light Sabbath candles last night."[9] I brought her to the Ark, which I opened to reveal the Torah scrolls. She then poured out her sadness that she couldn't light her electric candles on Friday evening because the bulbs had burned out. She said, "I lit them every Friday night for 98 years. Please, God, forgive me for not doing it last night." She then turned and ambulated back to her place. Later, after the service ended, another resident said, "We were treated to true prayer today!"[10]

These stories are samples of the spirituality I've observed and experienced during my tenure at the Charles E. Smith Life Communities. One could say they happen every day. The key element has been to create an environment conducive to prayer for people with moderate or severe dementia. It takes an investment of time, effort, and funds but the dividends are priceless.

Reference

Michaels, J.R. and Kozberg, C. (eds) (2011) *Flourishing in the Later Years: Jewish Pastoral Insights on Senior Residential Care.* Jerusalem: Mazo Publishers.

9 Jewish women traditionally light candles to usher in the Sabbath and Jewish holidays.

10 This and other stories about spontaneous prayer in long-term care settings can be found in "Promoting Spontaneous Prayer: The Blessings and the Challenges" (Chapter 9), Michaels and Kozberg (2011).

The Ministry of "Dedicated Suffering"

Mutual Spiritual Practice with Persons Suffering from Dementia

Dr. Jane Marie Thibault (Roman Catholic/United Methodist)

The experience of dementia is one of pain and suffering not only for the person whose brain is affected, but for all who are involved in their life—family, friends, and even professional caregivers. The anguish we feel when we witness the gradual fading of the light of cognition and recognition can be almost unbearable. We try to discover some meaning, but we're often left with "It just is what it is—a burden we have to bear." As primary caregivers, we may be tempted to ask such questions as "Is God testing my love, my commitment?" and "Why is this happening to him—a devout and dedicated person of God and family?"

When the illness worsens, life-long patterns of worship in a faith community may not be available to either the person with dementia or his/her care provider. The ill person may no longer seem to benefit spiritually or even socially from worship services. The caregiver often doesn't feel that it is "appropriate" to take her to services when her confusion increases and behaviors are distracting to others. Few faith communities teach members of their congregation how to welcome those with dementia (though they may sponsor support groups for caregivers). As a result, formal worship in a faith community is forsaken—often for many years. Also, as the disease lingers and progresses over many years, frequency of pastoral visits may become few and far apart.

Caregivers yearn for a way to participate with their loved ones in a daily mutual spiritual practice that could provide comfort for both throughout the course of the illness. For Catholics, saying the rosary together often activates memory and may provide solace. Reading favorite scriptural passages to the ill person may help until words are no longer understood. Beloved hymns—either sung or heard—may reinforce old memories of the presence of God. Pastoral visits (with or without communion) from faith community leaders may provide emotional support, especially for the care provider. But sometimes even the effort it takes to say a prayer together or watch a service on television is just too hard. This is especially true in the later stages of the disease, when the person is confined to the home or nursing home. When this happens, it seems that there are few options for mutual worship or spiritual practice. The act of being present to one another becomes sacramental, with the care provider carrying the weight of awareness.

Actually, there *is* a mutual devotional practice that can be helpful for both the ill person and loved ones from the onset of the disease until death—the ministry of what I call "Dedicated Suffering." This devotional practice answers three pressing existential questions:

- Is there an honest and creative spiritual response to the suffering and pain of the person who is afflicted with dementia?
- Can we care providers (family, friend, and professional) live a hopeful and meaningful life while suffering from two sources of pain—that caused by watching our loved one experience the ravages of dementia and that caused by our own physical, emotional, social, or spiritual pain we may be experiencing as well?
- Can we make meaningful, spiritual significance of our own and our loved one's suffering—even when s/he may not be aware of it?

If the practice of "Dedicated Suffering" provides affirmative responses to all three questions, just what is "Dedicated Suffering," how does one do it, and how does it "work"? First of all, it is a spiritual practice—an actual ministry—based on two powerful passages from the Christian scriptures. In Colossians 1.34, Paul asserts, "I am now rejoicing in my sufferings for your sake, and in my flesh I am completing what is lacking in Christ's afflictions for the sake of His body, that is, the church" (*New Revised Standard Version* (*NRSV*)). In John 15.5 and 7, Jesus states, "I am the vine; you are the branches. Those who abide in me and I in them bear much fruit… If you abide in me and my words abide in you, ask for whatever you wish and it will be done for you" (*NRSV*). Based on these scriptures, a very widely used devotional practice developed hundreds of years ago called "redemptive suffering," popularly known (and often derided) as "offering it up." It is not frequently practiced now, having gone out of theological style after Vatican II in the 1960s, but it has not died out completely and Pope Benedict XVI suggested its revival in

Chapter 40 of his Encyclical, *Spe Salvi*. When engaged in this practice, people who are suffering from anything—serious or just irritating—offer their sufferings to God who, in God's compassion, takes it and transforms it into help and loving kindness for someone else. It is very much like intercessory prayer, when you ask God to help someone else. However, a common complaint we hear from people who are in pain or suffering is that they can no longer pray—the suffering overwhelms their minds and they just can't concentrate on praying. In addition, the physical or emotional suffering may be so great that it edges out the experience of God's loving presence. This loss of God's presence, in itself, is another source of suffering!

I was introduced to the practice of "offering up" my suffering when I was four years old and confined to bed for six months due to rheumatic fever, which caused severe pain in all my joints and made me very whiny. My mother, a nurse, had no patience for whiny children. One day—when she must have been at her wits' end—she presented me with a small notebook and a pencil. She told me that whenever I was in pain and wanted to complain about it, I should "offer up to God" my pain for someone who was suffering more than I was, and she encouraged me to make a checkmark every time I did it. In those days the common theology had deceased souls stopping at a way-station called "Purgatory" to cleanse them of remaining traces of sin before being admitted to Heaven. Anyone who was still alive was encouraged to pray for them or offer up their own pain for the speedy release of the deceased persons' souls from the "fires of Purgatory." (Read Dante's *Purgatorio* for more detail about this state!) I was delighted by the thought that I could actually *do* something with my pain, so I eagerly got to work.

One particularly painful day, I checked 73 people out of Purgatory (according to my estimate) and told my mother I couldn't wait to die so I could meet all these folks I had dispatched to Heaven. Horrified, she suggested that I change my focus to living people who were suffering here on earth. We would watch the local news together in the morning and choose a story depicting someone in trouble or ill. We would then offer all of my pain as well as hers for the benefit of the person or people we chose. I loved doing it and thought a great deal about the people I might be helping (in those days I imagined Jesus sending down His Spirit—in the form of a dove, of course—to sit on their shoulders and offer them help). Most important, I found that focusing on others' pain made my own pain bearable because it was useful to others (and I stopped whining—clever

Mommy!). I've continued to dedicate what I now understand as my suffering energy throughout my life—including during a bout of Stage 4 non-Hodgkin's lymphoma in 2009—and have found that, in some way, it actually makes whatever suffering I am enduring more bearable. And I do believe it helps those for whom I dedicate the suffering.

Fast forward to modern times. In 1995 I was a medical school faculty member, a clinical gerontologist working with people suffering from various forms of dementia and their care providers. I found myself overwhelmed by the pain and suffering dementia causes for all concerned, and even thought about looking for different work, as I could find no meaning for this disease process and the havoc it causes. While praying for career guidance, it suddenly occurred to me that the practice of "offering it up" might be "resurrected" and modernized and broadened for use by anyone of any faith who was suffering from dementia, along with their caregivers.

To modernize the practice, I examined the essence of pain and suffering. These are the considerations that emerged:

- Some form of suffering occurs in everyone's life—it is the human "common denominator." We are free to determine how we will respond to it.
- Suffering of all kinds uses up—but also creates—an enormous amount of real, physical energy.
- Suffering makes us feel bad and often isolates us from others.
- We have an obligation to try to alleviate suffering, but in later life there is often "left-over" suffering that is resistant to treatment or palliation.
- If suffering involves an enormous amount of concentrated energy, which is usually endured, subdued, or avoided, why waste this energy? Why couldn't we offer the energy of our pain to God to use for another? If we don't believe in God, could we intentionally give our energy directly to another sufferer? When it is re-conceptualized as a potential gift for someone, one's suffering energy can have deep meaning for both self and for the larger community. Suffering energy thus becomes a gift one has the power and joy of giving, reestablishing one's role in society, relieving the sense of isolation from others.

There is conceptual/theological support for the idea that we can use our suffering energy for the well-being of others, the practice I now call "Dedicated Suffering." This support includes the following:

- Quantum physics asserts that all matter is energy and that we are all physically interconnected.
- Christianity teaches that Jesus is the vine—we are branches of that vine and Paul speaks of offering his suffering for others (Colossians 1.24, *NRSV*).
- Energy medicine researchers Jonas and Crawford (2003) write, "There is evidence to suggest that mind and matter interact in a way that is consistent with the assumptions of distant healing. Mental intention has effects on non-living random systems…and may have effects on living systems" (p.xvii).

How does Dedicated Suffering "work"?

Dedicated Suffering is very simple to do. If you are doing it as a caregiver alone, just imagine yourself taking your loved one's suffering, combining it with your own, and offering it to God, Allah, Jesus, Higher Power, Creator—however you envision that which is what I choose to call God. Ask God to turn this suffering into love or help for someone else. That "someone" could be another member of your family, your pastor, someone in your congregation, or anyone you know of who is suffering in the entire world. One caregiver I know checks the newspaper each day for a "cause"—a person or situation needing God's help. Once she decides on the "cause," she offers the suffering she and her mother with Alzheimer's are experiencing to God for that person. If you are non-theistic, you can choose to send the energy directly to the person who needs it. You dedicate your suffering energy once each day; you do not need to revisit it unless you want to. Often it helps to remember the person you have chosen.

In the earlier stages of dementia, when the person is still able to understand the concept of prayer, you might want to introduce this practice as something you can do either together or alone. If you are Christian, you might introduce it by saying something like: "Let's not let all this pain and suffering go to waste. St. Paul offered his suffering for the good of the people of the church. Jesus said that anything we ask, for His work in the world, will be done. Let's take the suffering this disease causes us and offer it to Jesus. We can ask him to turn it into His love and help for someone. Who do we want to be helped today?" The practice may be done after watching the morning or nightly news, with all the stories of death and destruction.

In addition to teaching people how to engage in Dedicated Suffering as individuals, I also gather people together in nursing homes, faith communities, and retreat settings to form ongoing Dedicated Suffering groups. In a nursing home setting, residents gather on a weekly, small-group basis, sitting in a circle so they can hear one another. Going around the circle, each person states the predominant suffering s/he is experiencing (in one or two sentences only). When all have shared their pain, they offer suggestions as to who should receive the gift of the combined suffering energy. Only one recipient can be chosen, so this can create lots of good discussion. Once the recipient has been chosen, they say a simple prayer: "Dear God (Allah, etc.), please receive our collection of suffering energy and transform it into loving energy for [name of person(s)] or for anyone You think needs it more! We thank you for this opportunity to share in your work of pouring love into the world."

When you and your loved one together (or you alone offering both of your sufferings) dedicate your pain for the well-being of others, you are actually engaged in a ministry as powerful as the ministry of prayer. The world needs this ministry. It is a way to stay connected to and concerned about what is happening in the "outer world." It gives profound meaning (and even usefulness) to the seemingly useless suffering that dementia brings.

References

Holy Bible, *New Revised Standard Version (NRSV)*.

Jonas, W.B. and Crawford, C.C. (2003) *Healing, Intention and Energy Medicine: Science, Research Methods, and Clinical Implications.* London: Churchill Livingstone.

Pope Benedict XVI, *Spe Salvi*, Second Encyclical Letter.

The material in this chapter was adapted from:

Thibault, J.M. (2004) *10 Gospel Promises for Later Life.* Nashville: Upper Room Books, pp.86–96.

Thibault, J.M. and Morgan, R.L. (2009) *No Act of Love Is Ever Wasted: The Spirituality of Caring for Persons with Dementia.* Nashville: Upper Room Books, pp.137–141.

Thibault, J.M and Morgan, R.L. (2012) *Pilgrimage Into The Last Third of Life: 7 Gateways to Spiritual Growth.* Nashville: Upper Room Books, pp.112–114.

BEYOND WORSHIP

Dementia-Friendly Faith Communities

A Church-Wide Response

Rev. Kathy Fogg Berry (Interdenominational Christian) and Gayle Hunter Haglund (Presbyterian Church, USA)

Each day, 10,000 people reach the age of 65 (Pew Research Center, 2010). For many churches, this means that a large percentage of your members are now, or soon will be, over this threshold. Economists and health care providers alike tell us that many of these people will live longer than ever before. This is a double-edged sword: On the one hand, with increasing life expectancy comes the exciting prospect of rethinking what aging means. Indeed, "vibrancy" is the new "aging." Yet, on the other hand, age wave predictions also include sobering facts about the increased likelihood of dementia, which will affect 50 percent of people 85 years of age and older. It is expected that, by 2050, nearly 14 million Americans will suffer from some form of serious memory loss, a three-fold increase from 2016 (Alzheimer's Association 2016).

Whole families are affected by dementia diseases, not just the person with the diagnosis. As the rate of dementia diagnoses increases, caregiving demands will rise along with accompanying emotional, physical, social, spiritual, and financial tolls. While these realities can remain invisible, hidden away behind the closed doors of individual households, communities of faith can learn to intentionally recognize need and discern a call to minister to families in life-giving ways. Literally millions of people stand in need of outreach and churches that will answer God's call to serve one another in love and faithfulness.

Unfortunately, few churches have recognized this deep and growing need. Yet the opportunities for spiritual growth are rich. As a church reaches out to people with dementia and their caregivers, opportunities abound for community interaction, intergenerational experience, and practical service. And yes, even for church growth!

To meet this tsunami of needs, it's going to take an intentional church-wide response. It's going to mean creating a climate where all are welcome, even if they might need to get up and pace or ask the same question repeatedly. Creating an open, safe, and accepting church environment where people can remain active members of their faith community for as long as possible is a worthy effort as we seek to reflect

God's abiding love. How wonderful it would be to nurture a dementia-friendly church where members experiencing these diseases could stay engaged and included and not feel isolated and excluded.

How can churches respond to this growing need?

Know your church members

Keep track and keep in touch. Taking note of church attendance is a critically important basic step in developing a ministry of connection to families coping with dementia issues. Does your church track family relationships? Do you note when family systems change, thus changing patterns in attendance? Community response relies on recognizing patterns and needs, even while respecting privacy and confidentiality. How can your church best convey true concern and track involvement in order to respond in love?

Create a safe and friendly environment

Consider inviting someone from the Alzheimer's Association to assess your church's facilities for safety and accessibility for people living with dementia. Challenges in physical ability, judgment, and sensory perception can lead to injury if the environment isn't carefully monitored for things which could prove to be dangerous. Rather than expecting someone with dementia to adapt to challenging surroundings, we can make necessary adaptations to anticipate their needs. Some things for consideration: Are ramps needed? Are there adequate railings on the steps? Is lighting sufficient? If you have a parishioner with dementia who wanders, does the church have alarms on its doors? Are bathrooms accessible and free of hazardous materials?

Collect and lend resources

One of the simplest but most powerful ways a faith community can respond is by providing a list of resources and a collection of materials people can access. Similarly, a small group of volunteers can meet twice a year to compile and update a list of organizations in your region whose services are dedicated to seniors. The list might include some of the following:

- Doctors and clinics specializing in gerontology

- Senior living organizations such as continuing care retirement communities, assisted living, memory support centers, and skilled nursing facilities. Each of these will be happy to provide materials for your collection, and an annual outreach can update contact information
- Your local Area Agency on Aging, Alzheimer's Association, senior day care centers, Meals on Wheels, Habitat for Humanity, Medicare programs, and state LeadingAge chapter.

Information is power, and often when people are overwhelmed and frightened they do not access information adequately. Systematically and intentionally gathering resources to share—and making people aware of your resource bank—is a tremendous service.

Another way to provide needed resources is to create a medical equipment recycling room at your church. As a family is ready to discard equipment no longer needed—shower chairs, electric lift chairs, grabbers, portable commodes—store them for the next person in need. Then, deliver the needed items with a healthy meal.

These are just a few ideas. The possibilities are many as we observe and listen. The more time you spend with those in your community who are living with dementia diseases, the more opportunities you will find to provide resources and meet needs that have been overlooked.

Offer instruction and support to members and your community

When Words Fail has created an instructional demonstration video and Study Guide for educating clergy, lay leaders, and caregivers.[1] This is best presented in group settings so that discussion can occur. Decide how often to offer opportunities for learning through coordination with your faith community's educational ministry. Perhaps you could sponsor a seminar at your church led by someone from your local Alzheimer's Association. Consider inviting neighboring churches to join you. For those who are unable to leave their homes to attend training, UsAgainstAlzheimer's offers a free teleconference series covering a wide range of topics with leaders in the Alzheimer's community.[2]

1 Available at www.whenwordsfail.com

2 www.usagainstalzheimers.org/alzheimers-talks

Ongoing opportunities for education about dementia and spiritual care are needed. As the members of your faith community receive information concerning dementia diseases and their effects, they will gain understanding and insight on how to relate to people better. Simply offering regularly scheduled educational opportunities will send a powerful signal to your faith community that your church is concerned and striving to understand the challenges of life with dementia.

Get involved in finding a cure

Each year the Alzheimer's Association holds community-wide walks to end Alzheimer's disease. Mobilizing church members to walk together can send a powerful message of love and support to caregivers and their loved ones.[3]

Learn about and then encourage congregation members living with dementia and their caregivers to consider taking part in clinical trials for dementia research. A clinical trial is a step-by-step process that studies or tests a new procedure, drug, vaccine, or device for prevention, treatment, screening, and improving quality of life. Such trials move research forward to find effective treatments and cures for diseases. Increasing participation in clinical trials for dementia research is vitally important, especially among minority populations.

According to UsAgainstAlzheimer's statistics, African Americans are twice as likely and Latinos 1.5 times as likely as white Americans to develop Alzheimer's disease. The Centers for Disease Control and Prevention reveals that, between 1999 and 2014, Alzheimer's deaths increased by 55 percent among all Americans, but they increased 99 percent for African Americans and 107 percent for Latinos. Encouraging church members to consider trials may make a true difference.[4]

Many organizations, including the Alzheimer's Association, Alzheimer's Foundation of America, and UsAgainstAlzheimer's, offer opportunities to add your voice to others at the local, state, and national level. ClergyAgainstAlzheimer's (a network of UsAgainstAlzheimer's)

---

3 Find details about when the Walk to End Alzheimer's is scheduled for your area by visiting www.alz.org/walk

4 The Alzheimer's Disease Education and Referral Center: 1-800-438-4380; Genetic and Rare Diseases Information Center: rarediseases.info.nih.gov; Alzheimer's Prevention Registry: endalznow.org; and the Brain Health Registry: brainhealthregistry.org

was created to promote dignity, compassionate care, and quality of life for individuals with Alzheimer's disease, and to provide support for families, friends, and caregivers, as we work together to STOP Alzheimer's by 2020. Consider joining the network and using your voice on behalf of those whose voices falter.[5]

Take stock of your church's existing resources

What is going on within your church that could be used to serve families coping with dementia? Chances are there are many existing resources that could be redirected to help meet the needs of caregivers and their loved ones.

- Perhaps your church hosts a scout troop interested in service projects. Why not encourage them to paint a caregiver's fence, bring over groceries, or, if appropriate, visit with a dementia patient?
- Do you keep an active list of members willing to provide occasional meals for members-in-need? Make sure that caregivers and members with dementia are on the list and adequately provided for.
- Do you have an active adult Sunday school or discipleship group that could be empowered to provide care? Put them in touch with caregivers to discuss how they might work together.
- Do you have prayer groups that could be enlisted to pray for people living with dementia and their caregivers, both within the church and the greater community? Provide them with a list of prayer requests that can be updated as needed.
- Are there service groups and service days dedicated to practical projects? Perhaps your faith community gathers to assemble school bags for children in need or kits for people facing medical treatments. Consider arranging for your memory-challenged members to participate.
- Are there singing groups or bands willing to perform as a full group or in small sections? Help facilitate a musical performance for members with dementia and their caregivers.

5 www.usagainstalzheimers.org/networks/clergy

- What about your nurseries, preschools, and Sunday school programs? Consider enlisting the children's ministry to write encouraging cards or draw pictures for members with dementia. Facilitate opportunities for young adults to be involved in ministry as well, perhaps by helping deliver meals or organizing participation in the annual Alzheimer's walk.
- Do you have a church bus or a list of people willing to drive members to church? Connect them to caregivers and establish regular routines to help those with dementia make it to services and other events.

The opportunities to use already-existing ministries are endless and unique to each church. Keep looking and dreaming, and encourage others in the community to consider ways in which they might use established programs and ministries to directly serve those with dementia and memory loss.

Provide congregational respite care

Looking for a way to support caregivers of people living with dementia? Your church could consider offering a respite care program. Respite means a short period of rest or relief. For your church, respite could mean providing several hours of care one day a month, once a week, or several days a week for loved ones and caregivers of people experiencing dementia. As your church provides a safe and secure environment, participants can enjoy stimulation and fellowship with new people in a place filled with God's love. For caregivers who are caring every day, both day and night, respite could mean time for rest and relaxation or taking care of business, errand running, or fellowship with friends and family.

First United Methodist Church in Montgomery, Alabama, is one example of a church which is successfully providing respite care. Six years ago, after enlisting and then training volunteers in dementia care, this church began a two-day-a-week, four-hours-a-day, respite ministry under the direction of church member Daphne Johnston. Since then, their respite program has grown to a four-day-a-week program involving volunteers from eight local churches and two synagogues. Each day 12 to 15 volunteers participate with an average of 25 attendees as they enjoy art, music, movement, intergenerational experiences, pet therapy, prayer, devotions, choir, service projects, exercise, and a host of other activities, including lunch. Most importantly, participants thrive from being together and building relationships with each other and volunteers.

More than 100 caregivers attend a monthly support group at First United Methodist, held while their loved ones are in respite care. Volunteers in this program average 1100 hours of service a year.[6] Your church can start modestly and build your respite program as needs present and volunteers are able.

Encourage and assist families in completing legal and financial planning

Establishing a medical and durable power of attorney and advance directive is extremely important for people with dementia diseases and their families. Your church might want to offer a seminar for the church and local community on legal and financial planning. Invite trained professionals to help. Most likely, people with this expertise are within your church's membership or can be easily found by a member.

When someone starts exhibiting memory loss, the need for families to do this kind of planning is acute. While the person can still make decisions for herself, it's good to get in writing what her desires are for her future care and who she wants to make decisions for her when she no longer can. It is always better for people to be able to self-determine rather than have other people's wills and desires imposed upon them during a time of crisis. When difficult decisions need to be made later, having the person's wishes in writing provides caregivers with the information they need to make decisions that honor their loved one. By providing information about financial planning ahead of time through seminars and other educational opportunities, you can help families avoid potential conflict or stress later, when the loved one is no longer able to express his wishes.

Provide support groups at your church or go with caregivers to outside support groups

Offer your church's facilities to the local chapter of the Alzheimer's Association for a new support group location. This could be a needed resource for both your church family and your broader community.

---

6 www.fumcmontgomery.org/respite

Some locations offer a group for caregivers while a group for their loved ones takes place simultaneously in a different room. Volunteers who have received training in dementia care could provide a music time, devotional, snacks, and other activities for people living with dementia diseases.

One available resource is *Seasons of Caring: Meditations for Alzheimer's and Dementia Caregivers* (Potts *et al.* 2014) and the companion *Leader's Guide for Seasons of Caring: Meditations for Alzheimer's and Dementia Caregivers* (Morgan 2015).

Keep in mind that some caregivers, especially men, are hesitant to attend support groups. Although they might recognize they could benefit from encouragement and conversation with people going through similar circumstances, the thought of going into a room full of strangers and feeling vulnerable may be too daunting. In such cases, you might volunteer to go with the caregiver to a group. He might be more likely to go knowing a friend is there with him. Over time, as he sees how valuable the sharing, input, and encouragement is, he'll feel confident to go on his own.

Throughout my work with families facing dementia, I've realized that an important form of support for spouses, in particular, is encouragement to continue enjoying and participating in what gives them joy as individuals. This balance is often difficult for spouses to find and may be made harder if they feel judged for their need to spend time with friends or enjoy activities that are affirming to them.

At Westminster Canterbury Richmond, a group of men meets regularly to support one another through the delicate and difficult balance of loving their wives through their journey with dementia and taking time for themselves. This group started with only a few men, but over several years it has grown to almost 20 members. As spiritual care providers, we may tend to focus most of our efforts on the person living with dementia at the expense of the spouse or other loved ones. This wonderful group of men reminds me to bear in mind the real needs of family members whose lives are deeply and permanently affected and who must be valued and affirmed as individuals whose lives we celebrate. Is there an opportunity to create a group like this one within your church community?

For those who find it difficult to leave their homes, but who have access to a computer, UsAgainstAlzheimer's hosts a confidential, online community group for Alzheimer's and dementia caregivers to share questions, tips, thoughts, and advice, while seeking the same from peers.[7]

Offer the joy of music through a choir or band created for a special purpose

Music offers an exciting and fulfilling arena for a church-wide response. Around the country, a number of organizations and churches have developed choirs for people with dementia and their caregivers. Dr. Mark Patterson, director of music at Salisbury Presbyterian Church in Midlothian, Virginia, noticed that even as several members of various adult choirs at the church began to experience dementia, they continued to thrive in the choir with small but thoughtful amounts of intervention.[8] One particular parishioner's experience astounded Patterson. "One of our chancel choir members with rather advanced dementia has been able to sing the Mozart Requiem in Latin and sing all of our repertoire. She still comes to chancel choir rehearsals regularly, even though she has had to drop out of most other activities in her life." Not only did Patterson find this amazing, it inspired him to pursue additional ways to reach out to others with dementia.

A presentation by Giving Voice Chorus at the American Choral Directors Association conference sparked Patterson's interest. Giving Voice Chorus is a program founded by Mary Lenard and Marge Ostroushko and developed in collaboration with the MacPhail Center for Music in Minneapolis and St. Paul, Minnesota. Lenard and Ostroushko both cared for parents with dementia and recognized the positive effects of music in their caretaking journey. The Giving Voice Chorus established its first chorus in 2014 and a second in 2016 for people with dementia and their caregivers and, through the Giving Voice Initiative, provides a toolkit for organizations who wish to start a chorus.[9] Patterson felt called to explore this further, as a natural extension of what his church was providing for a few people. He and his team have named this church's new choir, which will be open to members from throughout the region, the Joyful Voices choir.

---

7 www.facebook.com/groups/usagainstalz

8 The quotes from Dr. Mark Patterson and Joanne Sherman in this section are from an interview with the author, Jan. 14, 2018, Midlothian, VA.

9 Giving Voice Chorus, www.givingvoicechorus.org

Other churches experience success with such a choir. First United Methodist Church in Montgomery, Alabama, mentioned earlier in this article, offers the Side by Side choir for caregivers and loved ones with dementia. Sixty singers participate in this dynamic group.

Emerging research underscores the validity of music programs for people with dementia. The medial frontal cortex of the brain seems to link music, memories, and emotions. This cortex is one of the last brain regions to deteriorate in Alzheimer's disease patients. This may be why people with the disease can often remember, enjoy, and respond to music when other memories are lost.[10]

Professor Dr. Mary Mittelman at New York University's Center for Cognitive Neurology is exploring theories that music actually activates parts of the brain that dementia does not touch until the later stages. She founded a choir named The Unforgettables to study the effects of music on dementia patients. Further research is underway, but there can be no doubt that music groups such as The Unforgettables demonstrate the joyful effect of music and in coming together to sing (Musicoterapia Online 2013).

At the new Johns Hopkins Center for Music and Medicine, professors and students from the medical school and Peabody Institute are collaborating in multidisciplinary work that emphasizes innovation and community connection. Their early findings with the ParkinSonics, a choir formed for people with Parkinson's disease, demonstrate positive results. The Center is studying the effects that singing has on dementia patients and their caregivers, using a one-on-one model the Center calls "side-by-side singing." Their goal is to add more knowledge to a growing body of work on how music can heal (Byrne 2017).

The leaders of these choirs emphasize the importance of including a caregiver with every singer. This pairing allows for a shared positive experience and for adequate encouragement and assistance. Joanne Sherman, who directs Salisbury Presbyterian Church's Joyful Voices, cites another reason for the one-on-one pairing. "We incorporate rhythm, movement, and breathing exercises to enhance the experience and make a positive impact on physical health. And this will be much easier with a partner."

Receiving a dementia diagnosis is a frightening experience, and typically both the person affected and their loved ones are filled with dread

10 MacPhail Center for Music, www.macphail.org/impact-of-music/creative-aging

about experiences that must eventually be abandoned. "Participating in Joyful Voices is something they *can* do and something that the person with Alzheimer's or dementia and their caregiver can enjoy doing together," says Mark Patterson. Perhaps your church can explore ways to allow music to remain a joyful part of life for your members with dementia.

Just as participating in choirs can tap into musical memories and elicit joy from musicians living with dementia, participating in bands can help, too. For information and inspiration about forming a band containing caregivers, volunteers, and people experiencing dementia, look at projects like Music Mends Minds 5th Dementia Band.[11]

Allow members with dementia as much participation as possible within your faith community

Howard has been a deacon in his Baptist church for many of his 78 years. Now that he's living with Alzheimer's disease, he has trouble remembering things, and this Sunday, he forgets how to pass the offering plates up and down the pew rows. What used to be so familiar to him now causes confusion, and a look of panic settles on his face. Noticing this, his best friend, George, slips to his side and gently assists him. Once they reach the back of the church and the last pew, George helps Howard join the other deacons who are gathered to walk back down the aisle. They subtly help him, too, once they're at the front of the church, and thank him for his assistance. Howard returns to his pew with a look of contentment on his face.

For as long as possible, it is important to let people who are experiencing dementia continue to engage in ministry roles that have been crucial ways they serve people and God. Sometimes you may need to gracefully transfer them into another church role that you know they'll enjoy, while someone else "tries out" their old role for a specified time period. Often once they're in their new, less stressful role, they'll be relieved and not mind the switch. It requires creativity, diplomacy, and compassion. As you educate your faith community about dementia, they will become

11 www.the5thdementiadocumentary.com

more able to respond compassionately to challenging situations. Everyone will benefit from continuing to nurture one another, regardless of what physical roadblock seems to be in the way.

Invite affected families to participate in the life of the congregation

Make a special effort to invite families coping with dementia to participate in congregational events. Church programs, concerts, plays, preschool programs, and even the rehearsals for these events can be wonderful opportunities to help them feel included. Don't assume they will realize they are welcome—make a special effort to invite them through phone calls and notes. Perhaps you can help arrange transportation. Have extra volunteers ready and prepared to assist people as needed. If attending events is truly difficult or impossible for people, consider recording them and delivering a DVD to the caregiver so he can enjoy it with his loved one in their home. Regularly delivering a recording of services can be life-giving to those who cannot attend church services, should the caregiver not have access to the Internet. Even if caregivers can download content themselves, the value of a personal visit can never be underestimated.

Decide how to serve and then organize the effort

If your church is interested in forming a ministry dedicated to serving people experiencing dementia and their caregivers, start by forming a small group to examine options and resources and prayerfully consider ministry opportunities. Create a plan and methodically work toward coordination. Collaborate with other church communities and regional nonprofit organizations. It is rare for faith communities to actively and intentionally serve in this manner such that your church will make a true and needed difference. You *will* inspire others. But be realistic. Start small, see what works, and grow as you are able. Pray regularly for God's guidance and blessing. Trust God's Spirit to strengthen, sustain, and guide your efforts.

Pray

Never underestimate the power of ongoing prayer. Encourage your pastors, lay leaders, and congregants to remember in prayer those who travel the path of memory loss. Pray about those living with dementia and their families from the pulpit, during Sunday school, at prayer meetings, and individually. You've learned, evaluated, and considered. You've reached out and taken stock. You've prayed and felt a call to serve. You've recruited and organized. Now *act*. Step out in faith! Knowing that needs are deep, decide what your church can and will do. Likely you can do a few things well, but not everything. In Jesus's name, move forward! And keep track of your efforts, as this is a great encouragement for sustainability.

Share ideas with one another

We can help one another through sharing successes and challenges. As more churches begin to address the needs of those with dementia, we can learn from and encourage each other in the process. Please join us and share your community's efforts at our website.[12] "Therefore encourage one another and build each other up, just as in fact you are doing" (1 Thessalonians 5.11, *New International Version*).

Note: Adapted from a chapter in *When Words Fail* by Kathy Fogg Berry. Used by permission of Kregel Publications (etc.).

References

Alzheimer's Association (2016) 'Alzheimer's disease facts and figures.' *Alzheimer's and Dementia 12*, 4.

Byrne, R. (2017) 'Healing measures.' *Peabody Magazine*, Johns Hopkins University, Spring, 15–19.

Morgan, R.L. (2015) *Leader's Guide for Seasons of Caring: Meditations for Alzheimer's and Dementia Caregivers*. CreateSpace Independent Publishing Platform: ClergyAgainstAlzheimer's Network.

Musicoterapia Online (2013) '"The Unforgettables" chorus.' Comprehensive Center on Brain Aging, NYU Langone Medical Center. Retrieved from https://www.youtube.com/watch?v=7vSRk9Sbk1Q on January 17, 2018.

Pew Research Center (2010) 'Baby boomers retire.' December 29. Retrieved from www.pewresearch.org/daily-number/baby-boomers-retire on October 15, 2018.

Potts, D.C., Everman, L., Glazer, S.M., Morgan, R.L., and Wallack, M. (eds) (2014) *Seasons of Caring: Meditations for Alzheimer's and Dementia Caregivers*. CreateSpace Independent Publishing Platform: ClergyAgainstAlzheimer's Network.

12 www.whenwordsfail.com

The Dementia-Friendly Church

Rev. Dr. William B. Randolph (United Methodist)

Is your church dementia-friendly? The vast majority of older adults never experience significant memory decline; therefore, many churches are not overly concerned about being dementia-friendly. Moreover, people who have dementia are "out of sight, out of mind" because they often become homebound. Full participation in worship, activities, and special events by people with dementia requires special allowances by their churches.

It is important for churches to anticipate that some church members may develop dementia so that this illness doesn't rob both the church and members with dementia of significant relationships. The simple fact is, most church leaders do not even know if their church is dementia-friendly. Below are some ideas for helping your church become more dementia-friendly.

How to get started

Help the church staff, volunteers, and others understand how dementia affects a person physically, emotionally, and mentally. Understanding dementia goes a long way toward making a church more dementia-friendly. Training in the illness's progression and the various types of dementia is a great place to start. Invite representatives from the Alzheimer's Association to speak to the leadership team at the church council meeting or to the entire church during the midweek fellowship meal. While it is nice to have as many people as possible, be aware of what it takes to be a dementia-friendly church—the most important people to reach are the professional staff and key church leaders.

Five key areas are affected by dementia. Training should include how to design programs that take these five key areas into consideration:

- *Judgment*—for example, forgetting to turn off the stove or making irrational decisions

- *Time and spatial relationships*—getting lost or being unable to recognize where they are
- *Unusual behavior*—being agitated or fearful
- *Physical challenges*—having difficulty with balance and hand–eye coordination
- *Decline in sensory perception*—a decline in vision or hearing or depth perception; sensitivity to temperature.

Church leaders should not only be aware of the changes dementia creates, but also how to look for the characteristics of dementia. Such changes may happen quickly, and leaders need to be flexible if their churches are to be perceived as dementia-friendly.

Take action to become a dementia-friendly church

The next step to becoming a fully welcoming church for those with dementia is to evaluate the current settings and programs. Dementia caregivers and maintenance staff should do an environmental assessment. Involving caregivers in the process conveys support and acceptance. At the end of this article is a checklist for making such an assessment. Evaluations should include the following:

- *Assess physical settings*—look around the building for objects that could cause injury or be hazardous for those who have physical challenges, difficulties in judgment, or declining sensory perception. Identify areas of possible danger. Look for dangerous areas such as steps, HVAC (heating, ventilation, and air conditioning), kitchen, and restroom areas. Look at areas that might affect sensory perception—lighting, sound systems—and areas that might cause a fall. Focus on adaptations the church can make rather than expecting a person with dementia to make the adaptations.
- *Simplify activities and programs*—break up activities into simple, step-by-step tasks, and allow individuals plenty of time to complete them. Have extra help available for tasks that may be difficult for people who have dementia. Respect the dignity of all

by not asking dementia sufferers to do complicated or public tasks they are unable to complete successfully.

- *Support the individual's reality*—this is called validation. If, because of memory impairment, a person begins to live in an earlier life stage or forgets key details of his/her life, do not correct the memory unless the person is in danger. For instance, if a wife is looking for her husband who is deceased, do not correct her by saying, "He died a long time ago." Monitor behavior, especially the tendency to wander, and gently reorient the person with dementia to different locations or to the activities of the group.
- *Affirm individuals and their gifts, but note their limitations*—encourage church members not to condemn the mistakes of those with dementia, but to acknowledge they still have gifts to offer the community. Remember, the point of being a welcoming church for those with dementia is to prolong their active relationship within the body of Christ and to encourage their growth in faith with Christ. Yes, even those with dementia can still have a growing faith. It is okay to celebrate the relationship that has been, even if it is changing daily because of dementia.
- *Anticipate challenges*—it's impossible to prevent every problem from arising, but anticipating the challenges is important. For example, some who suffer with dementia are prone to wander, so providing alarms on doors is one solution. Another approach would involve covering doors that lead outside with a mural that looks like a bookcase.[13]

Put it all together

The final step in becoming a dementia-friendly church is to look for new ways to include those with dementia and their caregivers in the life of the church. The Office on Aging and Older Adult Ministry has resources to assist churches desiring to become more dementia-friendly. Many of our churches have older adults that currently suffer or will suffer from Alzheimer's and other forms of dementia, so preparation is important. Churches that desire to be dementia-friendly will begin to plan now even

13 The Alzheimer's Store, www.alzstore.com, is a source for products designed for people with Alzheimer's and dementia.

before they have a number of members with dementia present at worship and church programs. These churches will continue to seek better ways to minister to those with dementia. A list of a dozen ideas of targeted programs for those with dementia and their caregivers is listed at the end of this article.

Dementia-friendly church checklist

- ☐ Are all areas of the church clutter-free, well lighted, and mapped out or marked where they lead? Are there adequate storage places available for unused items? Is there a process for checking to make sure items are put away when they are not in use in public areas?
- ☐ Are classrooms free of complicated and misleading stimuli? Have you minimized background noise (radio, TV, computer, overhead speakers)?
- ☐ What are the expectations of caregivers when church members visit their family member who has dementia? Are caregivers' needs being met with support groups? Are respite programs available? What strategies have been developed to deal with the behavioral difficulties of those with dementia?
- ☐ Have you simplified tasks and directions so that everyone, including people with dementia, can follow them?
- ☐ In what ways is the church engaging with people with dementia to prevent boredom, depression, and agitation while they are present? In what ways are church programs helping members with dementia experience service to others, purpose, joy, and hope? How can the skills and abilities of those with dementia be best used during their time at church to give them a sense of being normal?
- ☐ What activities does the church offer that help to maintain the current cognitive function and spirituality of members with dementia? What new activities could a church offer, such as art therapy or dementia-oriented worship, which could be a family event?

- ☐ What role can the church play in preserving the history and relationship of people with dementia with other members of the church? (For example, recording their memories before they are lost.) What opportunities exist to help those with dementia continue to express who they have been in life? Do activity designs allow people to be remembered for who they are, and not for their illness?

- ☐ What is the church's "Plan B" for ministering to members with dementia and caregivers when they are no longer able to continue to participate in church activities? How will the church continue to minister effectively to, for, and with members when they become homebound or move to a skilled medical center?

- ☐ Have you completed educational programs and training for leaders about dementia? Have you taken into consideration the needs of church members with dementia and their caregivers?

- ☐ Has a careful study of the building and grounds been undertaken? Have the following areas been checked?

  - ☐ *Restrooms*—Have you set the hot water heater temperatures at 100°F or lower? Have you installed grab bars? Have you added textured stickers to slippery surfaces? Have you removed locks from the bathroom doors?

  - ☐ *Kitchen*—Is there a designated area for storage of cleaning supplies that is kept locked? Can electricity be turned off to the garbage disposal and any appliances when not in use? Are knives and other utensils stored in locked areas? Can appliances such as toasters, microwaves, and blenders be locked up or turned off? Can gas service to gas appliances be switched off when not in use? Or can the stove be connected to a hidden gas valve or electric switch, so it is impossible for it to accidentally be turned on? Is there a fire extinguisher nearby? Are the refrigerators cleaned out regularly?

  - ☐ *Storage areas*—Is there a plan to ensure that doors to storage areas are locked from the outside? Are tools such as drills, axes, saws, and picks locked up? Is there only limited access to large equipment, such as lawn equipment? Are all poisonous chemicals, such as paints and cleaners, locked up?

☐ *Throughout the church*—Have you disguised doors or set door alarms to the outside to prevent people with dementia from wandering? Have you removed or taped down throw rugs? Have colored stickers been applied to large windows and sliding glass doors? Have you removed poisonous plants or other items that might accidently get eaten? Is there sufficient lighting near doorways, stairways, and between rooms? Have you removed objects that block walking paths?

A dozen quick ideas to become a more dementia-friendly church

- Host Alzheimer's and dementia caregivers' support group meetings. Group leader training is available free through the Alzheimer's Association.[14]
- Offer a monthly respite time or day for caregivers of members with dementia. Include activities for those who have dementia besides sitting, sleeping, or watching television.
- Help people with dementia and caregivers look good by sponsoring a quarterly makeover day with area volunteers and cosmetologists.
- Offer a weekly or monthly special worship service for members with dementia, or designate special Dementia Sundays where the main worship service is designed specifically for those with dementia. Include familiar hymns rather than new ones in the service. (Resources are available from the Office on Aging and Older Adult Ministry.)
- Look for talents and abilities in people with dementia that they can develop and share with other people in the church. Affirm them in performing their service by acknowledging and thanking them before the entire church.
- Train church leaders and members in dementia awareness and strategies for dealing with potential challenges that might arise.

---

14 www.alz.org

- Offer a Memory Café (see "Are Cafés the Leading Edge of Older-Adult Ministry?" n.d.),[15] where the memory-impaired and their caregivers can gather to remember. Consider a workshop on making memory boxes for members with dementia and their caregivers.
- Have leaders of the church agree to and sign a code of behavior for interacting with members with dementia. (Examples of this would be listening patiently when members with dementia tell the same story over and over again; listening to what people with dementia are saying; avoiding correcting people with dementia when they do something improperly.)
- Offer a resource or reading center on dementia as well as a dementia newsletter with a review of some of the latest news on Alzheimer's. (This information can be obtained by joining UsAgainstAlzheimer's[16] and signing up for daily updates.)
- Develop a visitation team to visit members with dementia when they become homebound or move to a skilled medical center. Include regular Communion delivery and videos of worship services in the visits.
- Research, develop, and print a community resource guide for caregivers of those who have dementia.
- Develop a daily or weekly prayer chain and checking-in program for the families and caregivers of those who have dementia to minister to their mental, emotional, and spiritual well-being.

Note: This article was first published on the Discipleship Ministries website at www.umcdiscipleship.org/resources/the-dementia-friendly-church.

15 www.umcdiscipleship.org/resources/are-cafes-the-leading-edge-of-older-adult-ministry

16 www.usagainstalzheimers.org

Moving Beyond Name Tags

Becoming a Dementia-Active Congregation

Rev. Dr. Cynthia Huling Hummel (Presbyterian Church, USA)

People often drop out of their faith communities after a dementia diagnosis. Oftentimes it is the fear of forgetting names of friends that keeps someone home from services. For others, it may be the embarrassment of repeating stories over and over. For others, it is the stigma and the shame of the disease itself. For still others, it is the din and chaos of the coffee hour that causes dread. Sadly, this self-imposed separation can lead to social isolation, which in turn can contribute to loneliness, depression, and feelings of abandonment which can worsen dementia symptoms.

Thankfully, congregations across America are looking at ways to create a more welcoming experience for those of us living with dementia. Some congregations are asking all worshipers to wear name tags to help those of us with cognitive issues to feel less anxious about forgetting names and faces. This is a *great* idea, but I would like houses of worship to take the next step—to move beyond being dementia-friendly congregations to becoming dementia-active congregations. I have some ideas about how this might be achieved.

I am currently serving on the newly formed Tri-County Respite Care Task Force which covers Steuben, Schuyler, and Chemung counties in New York's Southern Tier. We are actively recruiting congregations in our area to offer "drop-in respite care centers" for those living with Alzheimer's and related dementias. Our task force is planning a conference to talk to area congregations about putting empty classrooms to good use. How? By providing respite care for exhausted care partners who desperately need a few hours of care for themselves and at the same time providing meaningful experiences for those living with a diagnosis.

It may seem odd to some that I am serving on this committee since I am a person living with early-stage Alzheimer's disease, but it makes sense to me! After all, I want to see faith communities move from "using name tags" to coordinating ministries that will help individuals and families who are dealing with dementia. And I would like to see more of these ministries in place before my family needs to access them on my behalf.

Through grants and partnerships, we are able to offer guidance on how to start a respite care program including providing volunteer recruitment ideas, offering assistance in how to vet and train volunteers, ideas about activities, nutrition, hospitality, record keeping, and more. We are encouraging small congregations to partner and "share the care." It might be that a program is housed in one place, but the volunteers come from different congregations. Or it might mean that the program moves from congregation to congregation. Both are good models. It just depends what works best for the community and the congregations involved.

Offering respite care is a great idea, but what else might congregations consider when thinking about a Dementia Ministry?

- Offer a space for an Alzheimer's care partner and/or person living with dementia (PLWD) support group. Encourage congregants to become facilitators!
- Start a "Memory Choir" where those with a diagnosis, along with family, friends, and interested folks from the congregation, gather to sing old familiar songs. Have a concert! Celebrate the joy of music and have a free will offering to raise funds for supplies.
- Invite PLWDs to participate in the life of your congregation and to help with tasks around the building or in worship based on that person's interests and abilities.
- Work with nearby clinics and hospitals and bring in trained medical personnel to offer memory screenings in your house of worship.
- Consider a Medical Ministry, where a trained nurse on your staff visits congregants in your house of worship, makes home visits to check on overall wellness, and makes referrals for additional care and/or services.
- Invite speakers from the medical community, the Alzheimer's Association, and other agencies to come to speak at your adult education meetings about topics related to dementia and care.

- What about starting a Caring Hearts Ministry, training volunteers to go into homes to be with those in the latter stages of dementia, so that a care partner might be able to attend worship or go to a doctor's appointment?
- Start an Arts Ministry for PLWDs and care partners in one of your classrooms! I participate in a once-a-month arts program. We paint, draw, work with clay, etc. It's great fun for PLWDs and for care partners. We even had a "gallery opening" and invited the community to celebrate with us. Remember, it's not about creating great works of art, but of creating a space of hospitality, creating memories, and having fun.
- A good number of people living with Alzheimer's disease are living alone. How can your congregation reach out to these people to provide companionship and care? Some no longer drive. Do you have a Transportation Ministry to help people get to your services or special programs? Could you invite them to special dinners? What else could you do to share God's love?
- Provide a dementia-friendly worship experience which is experiential, flexible, and mindful of sensory issues that are often present in those living with Alzheimer's or related dementias. For example, I cannot deal with a noisy, crowded environment or background noise. Why not have a "quiet room" where a PLWD can go when feeling overwhelmed by stimuli? Provide ear-plugs (I always carry my own) to help a PLWD cope with noise levels and commotion.
- Worship should include familiar elements—hymns, readings, prayers, liturgical practices—but may need to be scaled down or scaled back. Make sure that worshipers know that wandering is fine and that PLWDs sometimes will share their thoughts aloud. Be kind. Be flexible. Expect the unexpected. Experience the holy!
- Offer a special service of worship on September 21st, World Alzheimer's Day, and remember those living with a diagnosis, care partners, and researchers in your prayers. Take up a special offering to be used for a Special Dementia Ministry.
- Encourage people to sign up for clinical trials. The only way we will find a cure for Alzheimer's is if people sign up to participate.

Share information in your newsletters. Share information from the pulpit during announcements. Is there someone in your community who can speak about their experiences in a clinical trial? Invite them to speak to your men's and women's groups.

- Offer a special Bible study for those in the early stages of Alzheimer's, care partners, and friends.
- Participate in community activities that support Alzheimer's programs and services. For example, start a congregational team walk in the annual Alzheimer's Association walk or Longest Day fundraisers.
- Pay attention to legislation that affects families who are dealing with Alzheimer's. How will your congregation respond? What does the Lord require of *you*?
- Put your faith in action by becoming *more* than a dementia-friendly congregation—become a *dementia-active* congregation where everyone is welcome!

Blessings,
Rev. Dr. Cynthia Huling Hummel (PLWD)

BENEDICTION

That Which Endures

(Ret.) Bishop Kenneth L. Carder (United Methodist)

A friend whose wife died from Alzheimer's disease said, "Living with dementia is like having a perpetual funeral. Every day brings another loss until nothing remains but grief."

I can relate to the feeling! Since the onset of my wife Linda's frontotemporal dementia disease, life seems to have been one loss after another.

Dementia diseases gradually strip away memories, ideas, decisions, mobility, initiative, bodily control, recognition of family and friends, and finally breath itself. Each loss triggers grief, and the one you miss is sitting beside you. We lose them a brain cell at a time!

Of course, it isn't just dementia that strips life from us. Everything passes away—our looks, our intellect, our abilities, our energy, our mobility, our health, our independence, our cherished relationships, our productivity, and finally life itself.

Is there anything that survives through all the losses? Is there a constant which holds us together amid perpetual change, persistent loss, and death's finality? Or is grief all we have left?

Living and working among people with dementia has confirmed for me that one reality not only endures but actually thrives amid loss of cognitive and physical functioning. Dementia erases memories, strips away knowledge, garbles or mutes language, diminishes abilities, narrows relationships.

But this remains:

L O V E

The Apostle Paul declared it more than 20 centuries ago: "But as for prophecies, they will come to an end; as for tongues, they will cease; as for knowledge, it will come to an end… And faith, hope, and love abide; the greatest of these is love" (1 Corinthians 13.8, 13, *New Revised Standard Version* (*NRSV*)).

The expressions of love change, but the reality endures. I have known scores of people with one or more of the dementia diseases. I have yet to meet one who did not respond to being loved, even those who have been reduced to a comatose state. And even when the ability to express love is gone, love is generated with those who enter the comatose person's story.

Linda no longer comprehends the word "love." Yet, she expresses and responds to love! Language now fails her; but gentle touch, brushing her hair, a smile assures her of value and worth. She can no longer feed herself, so slowly placing food in her mouth becomes a sacrament of love. Mobility is gone! Turning her in the bed or smoothly transporting her to a recliner become means of bearing her in the arms of compassion.

She no longer has control of bodily functions. Washing her and keeping her clean is an exercise in love's humility and servanthood. Her filters are gone and emotional control is lost. Being with her, absorbing her anger and frustration with non-anxious presence, enfolds her in unconditional love.

The love is reciprocal. Linda's expressions of love are rarely verbal. Occasionally, she will say "thank you" to a service rendered. But her more typical expressions of love are these: a fleeting smile, reaching for my hand, raising of an eyebrow, look of recognition in her eyes, calling my name or those of our daughters, growing calm with a caress of her face.

Love is not sentimentalism or warm fuzzy feelings. It is entering the messiness, anguish, resistance, and hostility of the beloved with a non-anxious, gentle presence. It is action on behalf of the well-being of the other. Love is radical acceptance when behaviors feel unacceptable; compassion without expectations; continuing to care when the caring is not returned.

Love endures because love is God! The Scriptures clearly declare: "Beloved, let us love one another, because love is from God; everyone who loves is born of God and knows God. Whoever does not love does not know God, for God is love" (1 John 4.7, *NRSV*).

Love is that which is ultimate and the most permanent reality in the universe! Everything else may pass away. LOVE endures!

Contributors/Editors

The Reverend Cynthia J. Abrams
Former Executive Director of the Native American United Methodist Center
Director, Health and Wholeness Program
Special Advisor on White House and Congressional Affairs to the General Secretary
General Board of Church and Society of the United Methodist Church
Washington, DC

The Reverend Kathy Fogg Berry (Editor)
Chaplain, Westminster Canterbury
Richmond, VA
Author, *When Words Fail: Practical Ministry to People with Dementia and Their Caregivers*
www.whenwordsfail.com

Virginia Biggar
Director of Communities, UsAgainstAlzheimer's
Washington, DC
www.usagainstalzheimers.org

The Reverend Theresa M. Brion, MDiv
Chaplain, Goodwin House Bailey's Crossroads Falls Church, VA

(Retired) Bishop Kenneth L. Carder
Ruth W. and A. Morris Williams Distinguished Professor, Emeritus
The Practice of Christian Ministry, Duke Divinity School, and
Senior Visiting Professor of Wesley Studies,
Lutheran Theological Southern Seminary
Columbia, SC
Shifting Margins: www.shiftingmargins.com

Chaplain Drew DeCrease

Chaplain, Redstone@Home Hospice

Permanent Deacon, Roman Catholic Church

Rabbi Israel de la Piedra

Rabbi and Director of Spiritual Care, Miami Jewish Health

Rabbi, Mishkan Miami—The Jewish Connection for Spiritual Support of the Greater Miami Jewish Federation

Miami, FL

Robin Dill (Editor)

Former Director of Grace Arbor,

Congregational Respite Program of First United Methodist Church

Lawrenceville, GA

Author, *Walking with Grace Revised: Tools for Implementing and Launching a Congregational Respite Program*

robin.dill@comcast.net

Daisy Duarte

Patient/Caregiver Advocate, LatinosAgainstAlzheimer's Network

Springfield, MO

The Reverend Karen S. Dumey

Pastor, Westminster Presbyterian Church (PCUSA)

Cape Girardeau, MO

The Reverend Allison Draper, MDiv

Upaya Buddhist Chaplaincy Program graduate (2018)

Volunteer Hospice, No One Dies Alone, and on-call Buddhist Chaplain, Kaiser Permanente, Santa Clara, CA

Volunteer on-call and referral Interfaith and Buddhist Chaplain, Regional Medical Center, San Jose, CA

The Reverend James W. Ellor, PhD, DMin, LCSW, DCSW, BCD, CSW-G

Editor, *Journal of Religion, Spirituality and Aging, a Taylor and Francis Journal*

Parish Associate, First Presbyterian Church of Waco, TX

Professor of Social Work

Co-Director of the PhD Program in Social Work,
Diana R. Garland School of Social Work, Baylor University

Waco, TX

Author, *Aging, Spirituality, and Pastoral Care: A Multi-National Perspective*; Co-author, "Ministry with the Confused Elderly" in *Journal of Religion and Aging*, volume 4, no. 2 (1987), and *Tenth Anniversary Issue: Aging and Spirituality*;

Editor, *Methods in Religion, Spirituality and Aging*; Co-editor, *Aging and Spirituality: The First Decade and Aging, Religion and Spirituality: A Handbook*

Lynda Everman (Senior Editor)

Founder, ClergyAgainstAlzheimer's and WomenAgainstAlzheimer's Networks

Birmingham, AL

Co-editor, *Seasons of Caring: Meditations for Alzheimer's and Dementia Caregivers; Leader's Guide for Seasons of Caring; Treasure for Alzheimer's*

Help Stamp OUT Alzheimer's: www.facebook.com/HelpStampOutAlzheimers

The Reverend David J. Fetterman, MDiv, MEd

Chaplain, Redstone Highlands, North Huntingdon, PA

Hospice Chaplain, Redstone@Home Hospice, Greensburg, PA

Co-author, "Promoting Cognitive Health: A Formative Research Collaboration of the Healthy Aging Research Network" and "The Two Voices of Alzheimer's: Attitudes Toward Brain Health by Diagnosed Individuals and Support Persons" in *The Gerontologist*, June 2009, volume 49, no. S1.

Pastor Bobby Fields, Jr.

Former Program Coordinator, Alzheimer's Tennessee, Inc., Knoxville, TN

Pastor, Mt. Olive Baptist Church, Loudon, TN

Andrea (Yonina) Foster, PhD

Creator, Musical Memories

Activities Director, Jewish Federation Apartments

Williamsville, NY

Rabbi Steven M. Glazer, DHL DD (Editor)

Rabbi Emeritus, Congregation Beth Emeth, Herndon, VA

Principal, Glazer Consulting, Rockville, MD

Bioethics Faculty, Georgetown University School of Medicine, Washington, DC; The Uniformed Services University School of Medicine, Bethesda, MD

Member, Neuroscience IRB, National Institutes of Health, Bethesda, MD

Co-editor, *Seasons of Caring: Meditations for Alzheimer's and Dementia Caregivers*

The Reverend Nancy Gordon, MDiv

Director, California Lutheran Homes Center for Spirituality and Aging

Anaheim, CA

Jim Gulley, MA (Theology & Pastoral Care)

Member, Alzheimer's Association National Early-Stage Advisory Group

Pastoral Associate, St. Joseph's Catholic Church

Penfield, NY

Gayle Hunter Haglund
Director, Resource Development, Westminster Canterbury Richmond
Richmond, VA

Olivia Ames Hoblitzelle
Former Associate Director and Teaching Fellow, Mind/Body Medical Institute, Beth Israel/Deaconess Hospital
Dharma teacher, Cambridge, MA
Author, *Aging with Wisdom: Reflections, Stories & Teachings*; *Ten Thousand Joys & Ten Thousand Sorrows: A Couple's Journey Through Alzheimer's*
www.oliviahoblitzelle.com
www.tenthousandjoysandsorrows.com

The Reverend Dr. Cynthia Huling Hummel, DMin
Pastor, Presbyterian Church (USA), Elmira, NY
Artist and Alzheimer's Advocate
Member, Dept. of Health and Human Services National Advisory Council on Alzheimer's Research, Care and Services
National Early-Stage Alumni Advisor, Alzheimer's Association
Author, *UnMasking Alzheimer's: The Memories Behind the Masks*; *Glimpses of God's Grace: More Stories of Faith, Hope and Love*; *The Lord is Like a Firefighter*

The Reverend Bob Inkenbrandt
Senior Pastor, Gulf Coast Village Continuing Care Retirement Community
Cape Coral, FL
Volunteers of America: Our Ministry of Service: www.voa.org/worship

Amar Atma Singh Khalsa, LAc
Sikh Dharma International Minister
Staff Chaplain at Banner University Medical Center, Phoenix, AZ
amaratmakhalsa@gmail.com

Dharma Singh Khalsa, MD
Sikh Dharma International Minister
Founding President and Medical Director,
Alzheimer's Research and Prevention Foundation, Tucson, AZ
www.alzheimersprevention.org

Ek Ong Kaar Kaur Khalsa Michaud
Sikh Dharma International Minister
Teacher Trainer, Kundalini Yoga as taught by Yogi Bhajan
Founding Member, Ik Jot Foundation, Plano, TX
Director of Online Education, SikhNet.com, Española, NM

Assistant Director, Yogic Tools for Chronic and Critical Illness, Houston, TX
UN Liaison, SuperHealth: Yogic Science to Break Habits and Addictive Behavior, Española, NM
Author and translator
www.ekongkaark.com

Kirti Kaur Khalsa
Sikh Dharma International Minister
Co-founder and CEO, Alzheimer's Research and Prevention Foundation
Tuscon, AZ
www.alzheimersprevention.org

Sarb Nam Kaur Khalsa
Sikh Dharma International Minister
Executive Assistant, Office of the Secretary of Religion, Sikh Dharma International, Española, NM
info@sdministry.org, www.sdministry.org

Sarb Sarang Kaur Khalsa
Sikh Dharma International Minister
Chaplain, Presbyterian Española Hospital, Española, NM

Maria Khani
Educator and Public Speaker
Senior Chaplain, Los Angeles Sheriff's Department
Founder, *A Country Called Syria* Exhibit
Huntington Beach, CA

Truthful Loving Kindness
Assistant Administrator, Dementia Mentors, International Advisory Council Partner, Dementia Action Alliance, USA
California City, CA
www.truthfulkindness.com

Rabbi Cary D. Kozberg, DD, BCC
Rabbi, Temple Sholom, Springfield, OH
Founding Chaplain, Wexner Heritage Village, Columbus, OH
Founder and CEO of Side-by-Side: Life Transitions Coaching for the Later Years, Columbus, OH
Co-editor, *Honoring Broken Tablets: A Jewish Response to Dementia*; *Flourishing in the Later Years: Jewish Pastoral Insights on Senior Residential Care*

The Reverend Tim Langdell, MDiv, PhD, BCC

Board Certified Chaplain (APC/BCCi)

Ecumenical Catholic Priest and Zen Buddhist Priest

Abbot of Chaplaincy, Five Mountain Zen Order

Hospice and Palliative Chaplain, Roze Room Hospice, Los Angeles, CA

Co-author, *Coping with Vision Loss: Understanding the Psychological, Social, and Spiritual Effects*

www.Stilldaily.blogspot.com

Carlen Maddux

Editor and Publisher, *Maddux Business Report—Tampa Bay* (1984–2010)

St. Petersburg, FL

Author, *A Path Revealed: How Hope, Love and Joy Found Us Deep in a Maze Called Alzheimer's*

www.carlenmaddux.com

Rabbi James R. Michaels, DMin, BCC

Director, Pastoral Care, Charles E. Smith Life Communities

Board Certified Chaplain, CPE Supervisor, Charles E. Smith Life Communities, Rockville, MD

Co-editor, *Flourishing in the Later Years: Jewish Pastoral Insights on Senior Residential Care*

The Reverend Richard L. Morgan, PhD (Editor)

Co-facilitator, Alzheimer's Support Group; Hospice Volunteer, Redstone Highlands, North Huntingdon, PA

Author, *At the Edge of Life: Conversations When Death is Near*; Co-author, *No Act of Love is Ever Wasted: The Spirituality of Caring for People with Dementia* and *Pilgrimage into the Last Third of Life*

Greg O'Brien

Journalist/Writer, Cape Cod, MA

National Early-Stage Alumni Advisor, Alzheimer's Association

Patient Advocate, Cure Alzheimer's Fund, Boston, MA

Board Member, UsAgainstAlzheimer's, Washington, DC

Author, *On Pluto: Inside the Mind of Alzheimer's*

www.onpluto.org

The Reverend Linn Possell, MDiv

Dementia Educator, Consultant, and Speaker

Orlando, FL

Author, *Alzheimers: A Beautiful Spirit Celebrated*; *A Heart Full of GEMS*; *Dementia Guide for Communities of Faith and Leaders*

Daniel C. Potts, MD, FAAN

Attending Neurologist, Tuscaloosa VA Medical Center

Founder and President, Cognitive Dynamics Foundation (www.cognitivedynamics.org)

Medical Director, Dementia Dynamics, LLC (www.dementiadynamics.com)

Tuscaloosa, AL

Co-author, *A Pocket Guide for the Alzheimer's Caregiver* and *Finding Joy in Alzheimer's*; Author, *The Broken Jar* and *The Unlatched Door*

Blogger for Maria Shriver's *The Women's Alzheimer's Movement*: thewomensalzheimersmovement.org

The Wooded Path: danielcpotts.wordpress.com

The Reverend William B. Randolph, DMin (Editor)

Former Director of the Office on Aging and Older Adult Ministry, Leadership Ministries Division, United Methodist Church, Nashville, TN

Chaplain, Longwood Presbyterian Senior Care, Verona, PA

Elizabeth R. Reinert, MEd

Activity Director, Hillhaven Special Care Assisted Living Facility

Project Manager, Dementia Friendly Alabama, and Ombudsman Volunteer

Mobile, AL

www.caregiversunite.org

Chaplain Gillian Renault

Hospice Chaplain, Los Angeles division of Vitas Healthcare, www.vitas.com

Ordained in the Prajna Mountain Order

Los Angeles, CA

The Reverend Grace Schireson, PhD

Licensed Clinical Psychologist

President, Shogaku Zen Institute; Guest Meditation Instructor, Office of Religious Life, Stanford University

Palo Alto, CA

Author, *Zen Women: Beyond Tea Ladies, Iron Maidens and Macho Masters*; Co-editor, *Zen Bridge: The Zen Teachings of Keido Fukushima Roshi*

Pernessa C. Seele, PhD

CEO and Founder, The Balm In Gilead, Inc. (www.balmingilead.org)

Richmond, VA

Author, *Stand up to Stigma—How We Reject Fear and Shame*

Tryn Rose Seley

Photographer, Musician, Worship Leader

Scottsdale, AZ

Author, *15 Minutes of Fame: Empowering Caregivers of Those with Alzheimer's*

Norma Smith Sessions, LMSW

Former Curriculum Developer and Trainer, The Center for Child and Family Studies, College of Social Work, University of South Carolina

Chaplin, South Carolina

Co-author, *What You Need to Know About Me: A Notebook for Families and Caregivers of Persons with Alzheimer's Disease*

Jane Marie Thibault, PhD

Gerontologist/Clinical Professor Emerita

School of Medicine, University of Louisville (KY)

Spiritual Director, Workshop/Retreat Leader

Prospect, KY

Author, *A Deepening Love Affair: The Gift of God in Later Life* and *10 Gospel Promises for Later Life*; Co-author, *No Act of Love is Ever Wasted: The Spirituality of Caring for People with Dementia* and *Pilgrimage into the Last Third of Life*

Don Wendorf, PsyD (Senior Editor)

Retired Psychologist and Marriage & Family Therapist; Musician

Birmingham, AL

Author, *Caregiver Carols: A Musical Emotional Memoir*; Co-editor, *Leader's Guide for Seasons of Caring* and *Treasure for Alzheimer's*

Index

CPI Antony Rowe
Eastbourne, UK
June 20, 2023